Pathophysiology

made Incredibly Visual!®

Third Edition

Pathophysiology

made Incredibly Visual!

Third Edition

Clinical Editor
Theresa Capriotti, DO, MSN, CRNP, RN
Clinical Associate Professor
Villanova University
Villanova, Pennsylvania

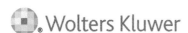. Wolters Kluwer

Philadelphia • Baltimore • New York • London
Buenos Aires • Hong Kong • Sydney • Tokyo

Executive Editor: Shannon W. Magee
Product Development Editor: Maria M. McAvey
Senior Production Project Manager: Cynthia Rudy
Design Coordinator: Elaine Kasmer
Manufacturing Coordinator: Kathleen Brown
Senior Marketing Manager: Mark Wiragh
Prepress Vendor: SPi Global

3rd edition

12 11 10 9 8

Printed in The United States of America

Library of Congress Cataloging-in-Publication Data
  Names: Capriotti, Theresa, editor.
  Title: Pathophysiology made incredibly visual! / clinical editor, Theresa Capriotti.
  Description: 3rd edition. | Philadelphia : Wolters Kluwer, [2017] | Includes bibliographical references and index.
  Identifiers: LCCN 2015046478 | ISBN 9781496321671
  Subjects: | MESH: Disease | Pathology | Physiology
  Classification: LCC RB113 | NLM QZ 140 | DDC 616.07–dc23 LC record available at http://lccn.loc.gov/2015046478

Dedication

For my first grandchild, Ethan Vincent Wolinsky

Contributors

Tracy Blanc, RN, MSN
Assistant Professor
School of Nursing
Ivy Tech Community College
Terre Haute, Indiana

Kim Cooper, RN, MSN
Dean, School of Nursing
Ivy Tech Community College
Terre Haute, Indiana

Stephen Gilliam, PhD, RN, FNP-BC
Assistant Professor
Georgia Regents University, College
    of Nursing
Athens, Georgia

Anabel Quintanar, MSN, RN-BC, CEN, PHN
Nurse Care Manager
VA Greater Los Angeles Healthcare System
Santa Maria, California
Nursing Supervisor
Lompoc Valley Medical Center
Lompoc, California

**Donna Scemons, PhD, RN, MSN, FNP-BC,
    CNS, CWOCN**
Assistant Professor of Nursing
California State University
Los Angeles, California

Julie G. Stewart, DNP, MPH, MSN, FNP-BC
Associate Professor and Director
    of FNP Program
College of Nursing
Sacred Heart University
Fairfield, Connecticut

Amy R. Weinberg, MS, DNP, FNP, AAHIVS
Nurse Practitioner
Stamford (Conn.) Hospital
Stamford, Connecticut

Wynona Wiggins, EdD, RN, CNE
Associate Professor of Nursing, Retired
Arkansas State University, School
    of Nursing
Jonesboro, Arkansas

Previous Edition Contributors

Kim Cooper, RN, MSN

Stephen Gilliam, RN, PhD, FNP-C

Phyllis Magaletto, RN, BC, MS

Susan A. Moore, RN, MSN

Anabel Quintanar, RN, PHN, MSN

Donna Scemons, MSN, MA, PhD, FNP-C

Julie G. Stewart, MSN, DNP, MPH

Amy R. Weinberg, MS, DNP, FNP, AAHIVS

Wynona Wiggins, RN, MSN, SCCT, CCRN

Contents

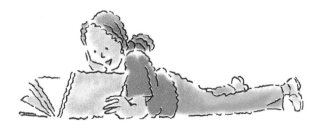

Chapter 1

The basics

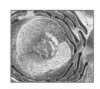

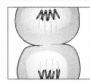

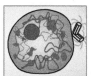

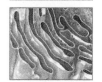

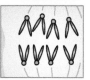

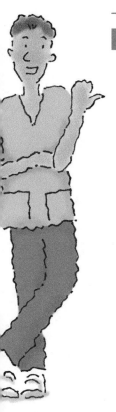

Cell basics

The basics

The cell is the body's basic building block and the smallest living component of an organism. The human body consists of millions of cells grouped into highly specialized units that function together throughout the organism's life.

   Large groups of individual cells form tissues, such as muscle, blood, and bone.

   Tissues form the organs (such as the brain, heart, and liver), which are integrated into body systems (such as the central nervous system [CNS], cardiovascular system, and digestive system).

Just your average cell

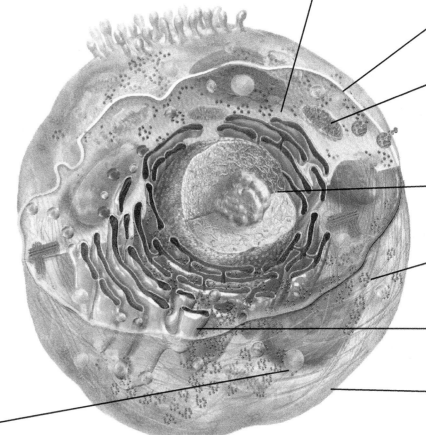

I am the gel-like substance that surrounds and protects the organelles

CYTOPLASM

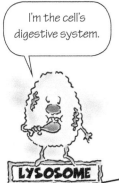

I'm the cell's digestive system.

LYSOSOME

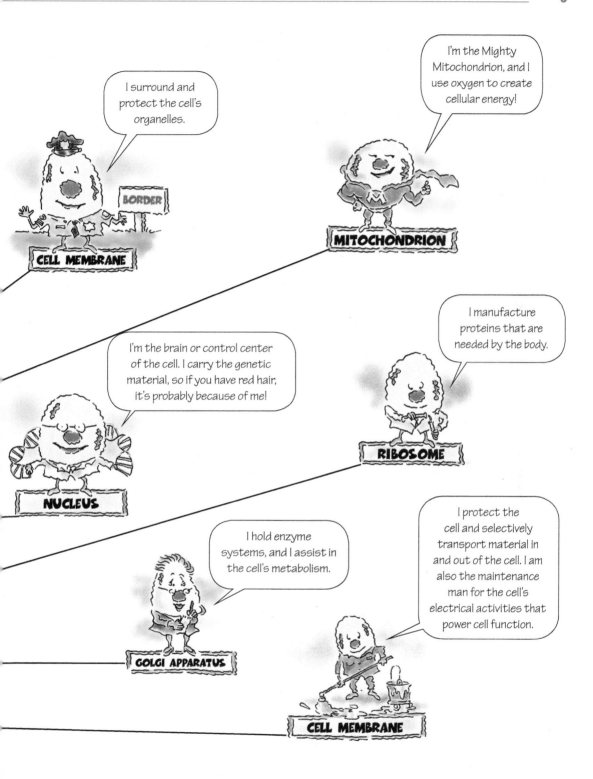

Cell division

Before division, a cell must double its mass and content. This occurs during the growth phase, called *interphase*. Chromatin, long filaments of DNA, begins to form.

Replication and duplication of deoxyribonucleic acid (DNA) occurs during the four phases of mitosis.

The great divide

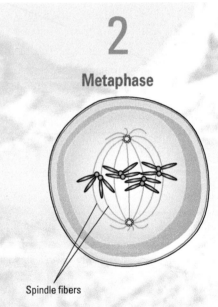

2
Metaphase

Spindle fibers

During metaphase, the centromeres divide, pulling the chromosomes apart. The centromeres then align themselves in the middle of the spindle.

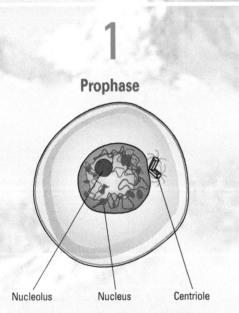

1
Prophase

Nucleolus   Nucleus   Centriole

During prophase, the chromosomes coil and shorten, and the nuclear membrane dissolves. Each chromosome is made up of a pair of strands called *chromatids*, which are connected by a spindle of fibers called a *centromere*.

3

Anaphase

At the onset of anaphase, the centromeres begin to separate and pull the newly replicated chromosomes toward opposite sides of the cell. By the end of anaphase, 23 pairs of chromosomes (46 chromosomes altogether) are present on each side of the cell.

4

Telophase

In the final phase of mitosis—telophase—a new membrane forms around each set of 46 chromosomes. The spindle fibers disappear, cytokinesis occurs, and the cytoplasm divides, producing two identical new daughter cells.

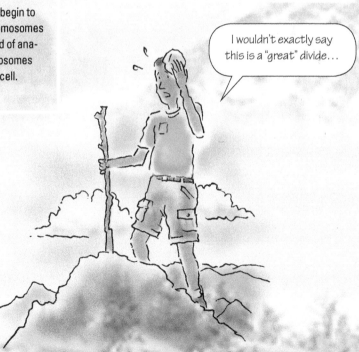

I wouldn't exactly say this is a "great" divide...

Cell adaptation

The cell faces many challenges through its life span. Stressors, changes in the body's health, disease, and other extrinsic and intrinsic factors can alter the cell's normal functioning.

Cells generally continue to function despite changing conditions or stressors. However, severe or prolonged stress or changes may injure or even destroy cells. When cell integrity is threatened, the cell reacts by drawing on its reserves to keep functioning by adaptive changes or by cellular dysfunction. If the cell's reserves are insufficient, the cell dies. If enough cellular reserve is available and the body doesn't detect abnormalities, the cell adapts by atrophy, hypertrophy, hyperplasia, metaplasia, or dysplasia.

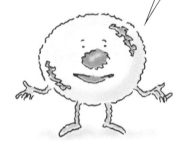

I guess you'd say I'm just your average cell.

Adaptive cell changes

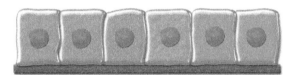

Normal cells

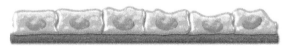

Atrophy
Atrophy is a reversible reduction in the size of the cell. It occurs as a result of disuse, insufficient blood flow, malnutrition, denervation, or reduced endocrine stimulation.

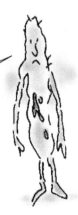

It appears I'm reducing in size. Well, at least this cuts down on my energy needs.

Hypertrophy
Hypertrophy is an enlargement of a cell due to an increased workload. It can result from normal physiologic conditions or abnormal pathologic conditions.

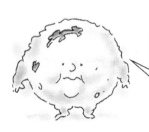

Uh... oh... I am going to need a lot more energy to keep these enlarged cells running!

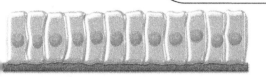

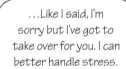

Hyperplasia
Hyperplasia is an increase in the number of cells caused by increased workload, hormonal stimulation, or decreased tissue.

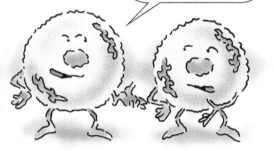

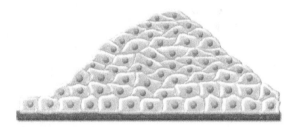

Metaplasia
Metaplasia is the replacement of one adult cell with another adult cell that can better endure the change or stress. It's usually a response to chronic inflammation or irritation.

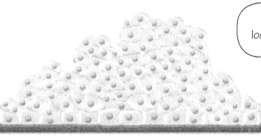

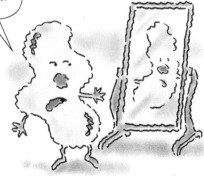

Dysplasia
In dysplasia, deranged cell growth of specific tissue results in abnormal size, shape, and appearance. Although dysplastic cell changes are adaptive and potentially reversible, they can precede cancerous changes.

Cell injury

Injury to components of cells can lead to disease as the cells lose their ability to adapt. Cell injury may result from any of several intrinsic or extrinsic causes and may be classified as toxic, infectious, physical, or deficit.

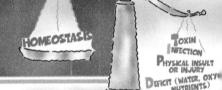

memory board

To remember the four causes of cell injury, think of how the injury tipped (or *TIPD*) the scale of homeostasis:

HOMEOSTASIS

TOXIN
INFECTION
PHYSICAL INSULT OR INJURY
DEFICIT (WATER, OXY... NUTRIENTS)

Toxic injury

Toxic injuries may be caused by factors inside the body (endogenous factors) or outside the body (exogenous factors). Common endogenous factors include genetically determined metabolic errors, gross malformations, and hypersensitivity reactions. Exogenous factors include alcohol, lead, carbon monoxide, cigarette smoke, pesticides, carcinogens, chemotherapeutic agents, and immunosuppressive drugs.

Deficit injury

When a deficit of water, oxygen, or nutrients occurs or if constant temperature and adequate waste disposal aren't maintained, cellular synthesis can't take place. A lack of just one of these basic requirements can cause cell disruption or death.

Physical injury

Physical injury results from a disruption in the cell or in the relationships of the intracellular organelles (such as mitochondria, nuclei, lysosomes, and ribosomes). Two major types of physical injury are thermal (electrical or radiation) and mechanical (trauma or surgery).

Infectious injury

Viral, fungal, protozoal, and bacterial organisms can cause cell injury or death. These organisms affect cell integrity, usually by interfering with cell synthesis, producing mutant cells. For example, human immunodeficiency virus (HIV) kills T cells and inserts its own RNA into the T-cell DNA. Then the T cell cannot defend the body anymore and acts as a factory for making more HIV.

Brrr! Frostbite can d-d-damage cells and cause ph-ph-physical injury and p-p-pain.

I hate to give you up, but I think it's time. Your carbon monoxide emissions are way beyond healthy.

We can do a lot of damage by interfering with cell synthesis, which can kill the cell or produce mutant cells that don't function properly anymore.

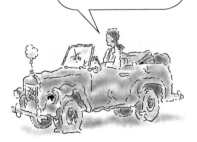

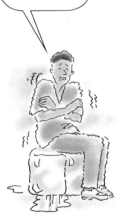

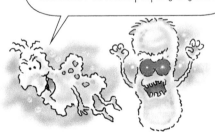

Stress and disease

When a stressor such as a life change occurs, a person can respond in one of two ways—by adapting successfully or by failing to adapt. A maladaptive response to stress may result in disease. The underlying stressor may be real or perceived.

Hans Selye, a pioneer in the study of stress and disease, described stages of adaptation to a stressful event: alarm, resistance, and exhaustion or recovery. The stress response is controlled by actions taking place in the nervous and endocrine systems. These actions try to redirect energy to the organ—such as the heart, lungs, or brain—that's most affected by the stress.

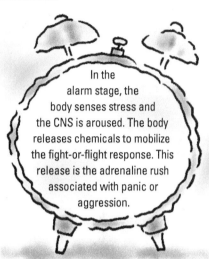

In the alarm stage, the body senses stress and the CNS is aroused. The body releases chemicals to mobilize the fight-or-flight response. This release is the adrenaline rush associated with panic or aggression.

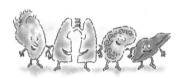

When stress strikes

According to Hans Selye's General Adaptation Model, the body reacts to stress in the stages depicted here.

In the resistance stage, the body either adapts and achieves homeostasis or fails to adapt and enters the exhaustion stage, resulting in disease.

Physical or psychological stressor

Alarm reaction
• Arousal of the CNS begins.   • Epinephrine, norepinephrine, and cortisol are released, causing an increase in heart rate, oxygen intake, and mental activity and increased force of heart contractions.

Resistance
• The body responds to the stressor and attempts to return to homeostasis.   • Coping mechanisms, such as avoidance or sublimation, are used.

Recovery	Exhaustion
	• The body can no longer produce hormones such as in the alarm stage. • Organ damage begins.

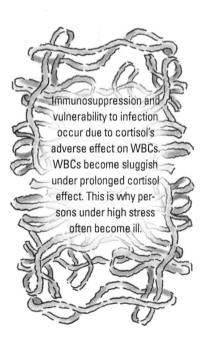

Immunosuppression and vulnerability to infection occur due to cortisol's adverse effect on WBCs. WBCs become sluggish under prolonged cortisol effect. This is why persons under high stress often become ill.

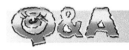

Able to label?

Label the parts of a cell indicated in this illustration.

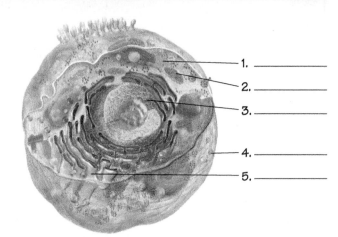

1. _____

2. _____

3. _____

4. _____

5. _____

Show and tell

Identify the four phases of mitosis shown in these illustrations, and explain what happens in each phase.

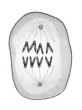 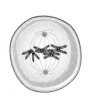 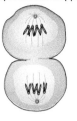 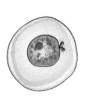

1. _____   2. _____   3. _____   4. _____

Answers: Able to label? 1. cytoplasm, 2. mitochondrion, 3. nucleus, 4. ribosome, 5. Golgi apparatus Show and tell 1. anaphase; centromeres separate and pull replicated chromosomes toward opposite sides of the cell, 2. metaphase; centromeres divide, pulling chromosomes apart, 3. telophase; final phase of mitosis; produces two identical new daughter cells, 4. prophase; chromosomes coil and shorten, and the nuclear membrane dissolves.

Selected References

Barrett, K., Barman, S., Boitano, S., & Brooks, H. (2012). *Ganong's review of medical physiology* (24th ed.). New York, NY: McGraw-Hill.

Hall, J. (2011). *Guyton & Hall textbook of medical physiology* (12th ed.). Philadelphia, PA: Elsevier.

Harvey, R. A., & Ferrier, D. R. (2013). *Lippincott's illustrated reviews: Biochemistry* (6th ed.). Philadelphia, PA: Wolters Kluwer.

Kumar, V., Abbas, A. K., & Aster, J. C. (2015). *Robbins & Cotran's pathologic basis of disease* (9th ed.). Philadelphia, PA: Elsevier-Saunders.

Nature. (2014a). Human genome collection. Retrieved from: http://www.nature.com/nature/supplements/collections/humangenome/ on June 12, 2015.

Nature. (2014b). Senescence, ageing and cancer. Retrieved from: http://www.nature.com/nature/focus/senescence/ on June 15, 2015.

U.S. Department of Energy. (2014). Human Genome Project information. Retrieved from: http://web.ornl.gov/sci/techresources/Human_Genome/index.shtm on June 17, 2015.

Chapter 2

Cardiovascular disorders

 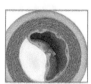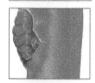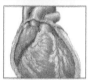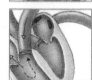
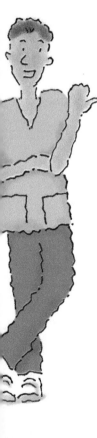

Acute coronary syndromes

Cardiovascular disorders

Acute myocardial infarction (MI), including ST-segment elevation MI and non-ST-segment elevation MI, and unstable angina are part of a group of diseases called *acute coronary syndrome* (ACS).

How it happens

1. Plaque in the coronary arteries ruptures or erodes.
2. Platelets adhere to damaged area and become exposed to activating factors (collagen, thrombin, von Willebrand factor).
3. Platelet activation produces glycoprotein IIb and IIIa receptors that bind fibrinogen.
4. Platelet aggregation and adhesion continue, enlarging the thrombus.
5. ECG shows ST elevation as in myocardial infarction.

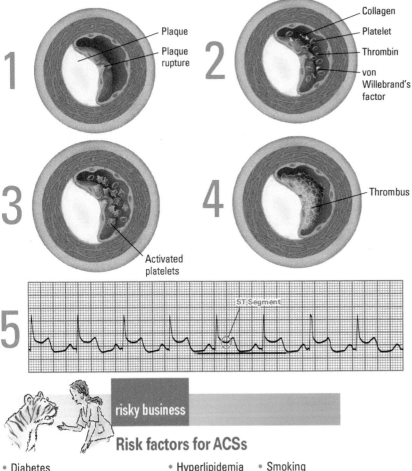

1 — Plaque, Plaque rupture

2 — Collagen, Platelet, Thrombin, von Willebrand's factor

3 — Activated platelets

4 — Thrombus

5 — ST Segment

risky business

Risk factors for ACSs

- Diabetes
- Obesity
- Family history of heart disease
- High-fat, high-carbohydrate diet
- Hyperlipidemia
- Hypertension
- Menopause
- Smoking
- Stress
- Lack of exercise

What to look for

MI

- Chest pain (severe, persistent, squeezing, or crushing)
  - Usually in substernal chest
  - May radiate to the left arm, neck, jaw, or shoulder blade
  - Unrelieved by rest or nitroglycerin
- Perspiration
- Anxiety
- Feeling of impending doom
- Fatigue
- Shortness of breath
- Hypotension
- Nausea and vomiting

Unstable angina

- Chest pain (burning, squeezing, or crushing)
  - Usually in the substernal chest
  - May radiate to the left arm, neck, jaw, or shoulder blade
  - Relieved by nitroglycerin

Atypical chest pain

Women may experience chest pain typically associated with acute ischemia and MI; however, women—and occasionally men, elderly patients, and patients with diabetes—may also experience atypical chest pain. Signs and symptoms of atypical chest pain include the following:

- Upper back discomfort between the shoulder blades
- Palpitations
- A feeling of fullness in the neck
- Nausea
- Abdominal discomfort
- Dizziness
- Unexplained fatigue
- Exhaustion or shortness of breath

Tissue destruction in MI

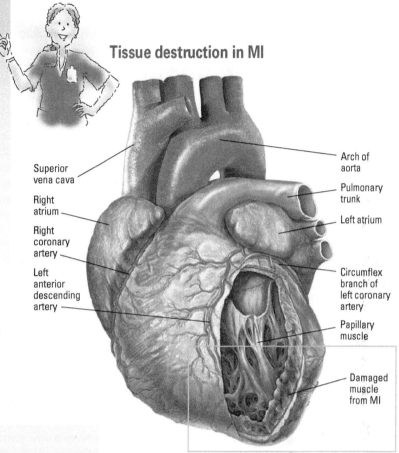

Superior vena cava

Right atrium

Right coronary artery

Left anterior descending artery

Arch of aorta

Pulmonary trunk

Left atrium

Circumflex branch of left coronary artery

Papillary muscle

Damaged muscle from MI

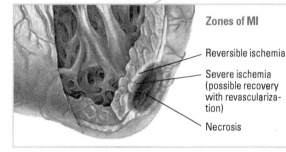

Zones of MI

Reversible ischemia

Severe ischemia (possible recovery with revascularization)

Necrosis

Aortic aneurysm

An aortic aneurysm (AA) is an abnormal dilation in the aortic arterial wall. An aneurysm generally occurs between the renal arteries and iliac branches. In a saccular aneurysm, an outpouching occurs in the arterial wall. In fusiform aneurysms, the outpouching appears spindle shaped and encompasses the entire aortic circumference. In a false aneurysm, the outpouching occurs when the entire vessel wall is injured and leads to a sac formation affecting the artery or heart.

How it happens

1. Degenerative changes create a focal weakness in the muscular layer of the aorta.
2. The inner and outer layers stretch outward to create a bulge, called an *aneurysm*.
3. Pressure from the blood pulsing through the aorta weakens the vessel wall and enlarges the aneurysm.

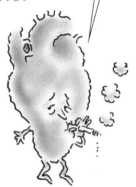

risky business

Risk factors for AA

- Long-standing hypertension
- Older adult male over age 65
- Smoking/tobacco use
- Arteriosclerosis in another area of the body
- Family history

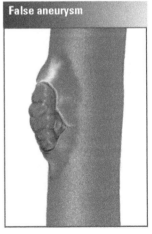

I've got hypertension, too. It's not looking good for me, is it?

Types of aneurysms

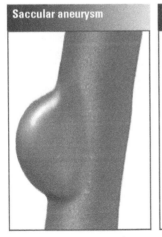

Saccular aneurysm

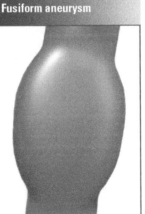

Fusiform aneurysm

False aneurysm

Dissecting aneurysm

Aneurysms can dissect or rip when bleeding into the weakened artery causes the artery wall to split.

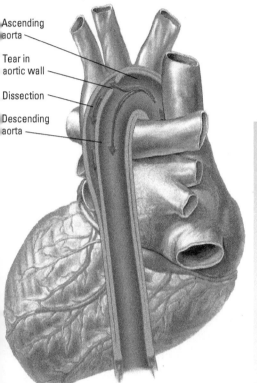

Ascending aorta

Tear in aortic wall

Dissection

Descending aorta

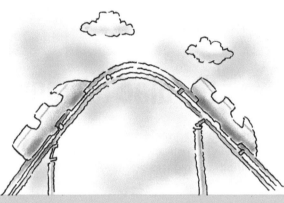

What to look for

Ascending aortic aneurysm
* Pain
* Bradycardia
* Murmur of aortic insufficiency
* Pericardial friction rub
* Unequal carotid and radial pulses
* Different blood pressures in right and left arms

Descending aortic aneurysm
* Pain (suddenly between shoulder blades and chest)
* Hoarseness
* Dyspnea and stridor
* Dysphagia
* Dry cough

Abdominal aortic aneurysm
* Systolic bruit over aorta
* Tenderness on deep palpation
* Lumbar pain radiating to flank and groin
* Wide aortic pulsation palpable in abdomen
* Commonly asymptomatic until rupture

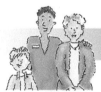

age-old story

Age alert for AA

Ascending AAs are usually seen in hypertensive men younger than age 60.

Descending AAs may occur in young patients after a traumatic chest injury or after infection but are most common in elderly men with hypertension.

Cardiac tamponade

Cardiac tamponade is a rapid, unchecked increase in pressure due to fluid accumulation in the pericardial sac. This compresses the heart, impairs diastolic filling, and reduces cardiac output.

How it happens

Cardiac tamponade usually results from blood or fluid that accumulates in the pericardial sac and compresses the heart. This compression obstructs blood flow to the ventricles and reduces the amount of blood pumped out of the heart with each contraction. Possible causes include recent heart surgery, MI, pericarditis from bacterial or viral infection, cardiac trauma, or malignant effusions.

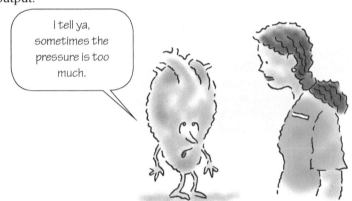

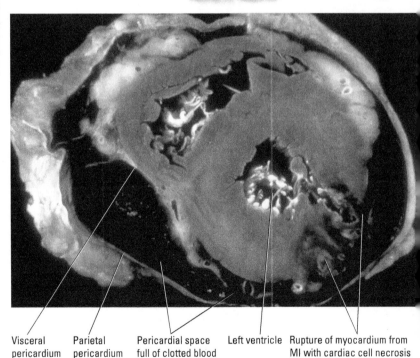

Visceral pericardium   Parietal pericardium   Pericardial space full of clotted blood   Left ventricle   Rupture of myocardium from MI with cardiac cell necrosis

What to look for

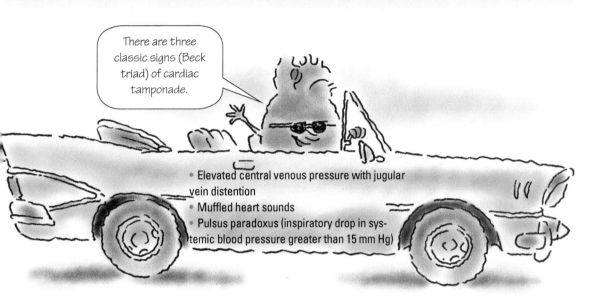

There are three classic signs (Beck triad) of cardiac tamponade.

- Elevated central venous pressure with jugular vein distention
- Muffled heart sounds
- Pulsus paradoxus (inspiratory drop in systemic blood pressure greater than 15 mm Hg)

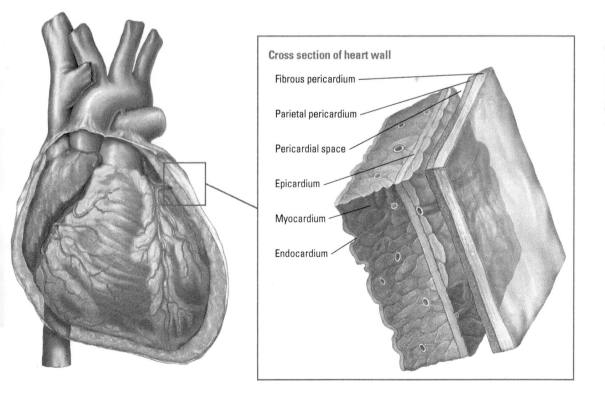

Cross section of heart wall

Fibrous pericardium

Parietal pericardium

Pericardial space

Epicardium

Myocardium

Endocardium

Cardiogenic shock

Cardiogenic shock is a commonly fatal complication of various acute and chronic disorders that impair the heart's ability to maintain adequate tissue perfusion. It can result from any condition that causes significant left ventricular dysfunction and reduced cardiac output, with the most common cause being acute MI. Cardiogenic shock is a severe type of heart failure.

How it happens

Cycle of decompensation

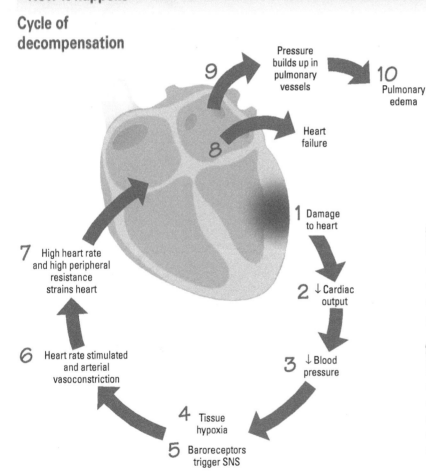

9 Pressure builds up in pulmonary vessels

10 Pulmonary edema

8 Heart failure

1 Damage to heart

7 High heart rate and high peripheral resistance strains heart

2 ↓ Cardiac output

6 Heart rate stimulated and arterial vasoconstriction

3 ↓ Blood pressure

4 Tissue hypoxia

5 Baroreceptors trigger SNS

What to look for

- Cyanotic mucous membranes
- Cool, clammy skin
- Weak, thready pulse
- Delayed capillary refill
- Shortness of breath
- Pallor
- Decreased level of consciousness

INCREASED

- Heart rate
- Respiration
- Pulmonary capillary wedge pressure

DECREASED

- Systolic pressure (<80 mm Hg)
- Urine output (<20 mL/hour)
- Oxygen saturation
- Left ventricular ejection fraction
- Stroke volume

Cardiomyopathy

Dilated

Dilated cardiomyopathy is a disease due to weakened heart muscle fibers. It usually isn't diagnosed until it has reached an advanced stage and the prognosis is generally poor.

How it happens

Dilated cardiomyopathy results from damage to cardiac muscle fibers. The resulting loss of muscle tone grossly dilates all four chambers of the heart, giving the heart a globular shape.

What to look for

- Shortness of breath
- Orthopnea
- Dyspnea on exertion
- Fatigue
- Dry cough at night
- Peripheral edema
- Hepatomegaly
- Jugular vein distention
- Weight gain
- Peripheral cyanosis
- Tachycardia
- Pansystolic murmur
- S_3 and S_4 gallop rhythms
- Irregular pulse
- Decreased renal function

7

5

4

6

1

3

2

Atria become dilated causing atrial fibrillation.

Papillary muscles of the ventricles stretched by excess blood volume.

Mitral and tricuspid valves do not close tightly.

Blood accumulates in the atria and stretch out the atria.

The cycle begins

Poor cardiac muscle strength causes left-sided and right-sided heart failure.

Low cardiac output pushed forward into the aorta.

High amount of blood volume accumulates in the left and right ventricles.

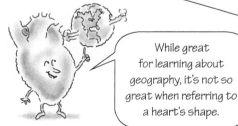

While great for learning about geography, it's not so great when referring to a heart's shape.

Cardiomyopathy

Hypertrophic

Hypertrophic cardiomyopathy is a common genetic disease of the heart that is characterized by unexplained LV hypertrophy, particularly an enlarged interventricular septum. It mainly limits filling of the ventricles during diastole.

How it happens

About 50% of the time, hypertrophic cardiomyopathy is transmitted as an autosomal dominant trait. Other causes aren't known.

The damage is done

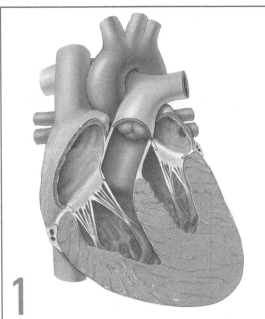

1 The left ventricle and interventricular septum hypertrophy and become stiff, noncompliant, and unable to relax during ventricular filling.

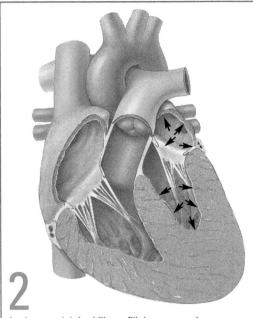

2 As the ventricle's ability to fill decreases, the pressure increases, and left atrial and pulmonary venous pressures rise.

Fifty percent of all sudden deaths in competitive athletes are caused by hypertrophic obstructive cardiomyopathy. Good enough reason for me to get a preparticipation athletic physical exam!

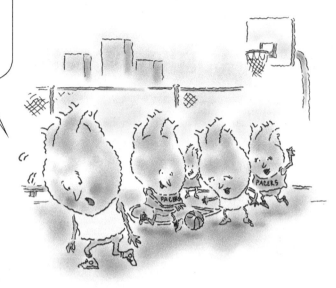

What to look for

- Chest discomfort, particularly with exercise.
- A majority of patients are asymptomatic.
- Systolic ejection murmur along the left sternal border and at the apex.
- Angina with exertion.
- Syncope (fainting).
- Activity intolerance.
- Irregular pulse (atrial fibrillation).

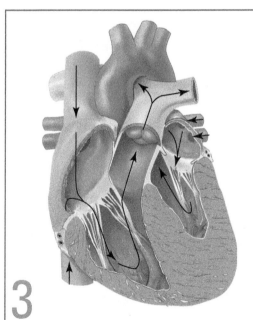

3

The left ventricle forcefully contracts but can't sufficiently relax.

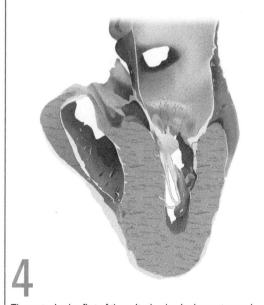

4

The anterior leaflet of the mitral valve is drawn toward the interventricular septum as the blood is forcefully ejected. Early closure of the outflow tract results because of the decreasing ejection fraction.

Cardiomyopathy

Restrictive

Restrictive cardiomyopathy is a disease of heart muscle fibers. Commonly, it is caused by long-standing hypertension that causes the left ventricle to hypertrophy.

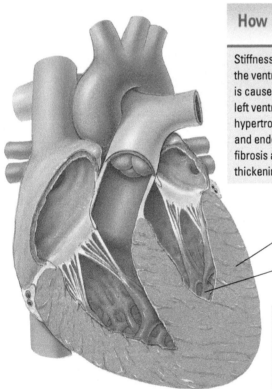

Left ventricular hypertrophy

Decreased ventricular chamber size

How it happens

Stiffness of the ventricle is caused by left ventricular hypertrophy and endocardial fibrosis and thickening.

This stiffness reduces the ventricle's ability to relax and fill during diastole.

The rigid myocardium fails to contract completely during systole.

As a result, cardiac output falls.

What to look for

- Hypertension
- Fatigue
- Dyspnea
- Orthopnea
- Chest pain
- Edema
- Liver engorgement
- Peripheral cyanosis
- Irregular heart rate
- Pallor
- S_3 or S_4 gallop rhythm

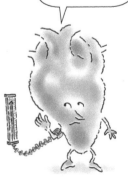

Good reason to make me have my BP checked often.

Coronary artery disease

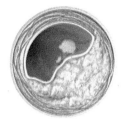

If excessive amounts of fat circulate in the blood, fatty deposits (called *plaques*) can accumulate in the arteries. This buildup, called *atherosclerosis*, causes the vessels to narrow or become obstructed. Arteriosclerotic plaque can also break apart, and pieces can become *emboli* that lodge in distal arteries and arterioles.

How it happens

Coronary artery disease (CAD) results when atherosclerotic plaque fills the lumens of the coronary arteries and obstructs blood flow to the heart, diminishing the supply of oxygen and nutrients to the heart tissue.

What to look for

- Angina (chest pain)
- Nausea and vomiting
- Cool extremities
- Diaphoresis
- Pallor
- Dyspnea on exertion

risky business

Risk factors for CAD

Rising low-density lipoprotein (LDL) and triglyceride levels—LDLs should be less than 100 mg/dL and triglycerides less than 150 mg/dL.

Inadequate control of hypertension, diabetes, and obesity; diet, exercise, and lifestyle changes are key to treating this condition.

Sex—CAD is more common in men over age 45 and women over age 55.

Kinfolk—Heredity is a nonmodifiable risk factor.

Smoking—The sooner stopped, the better.

Coronary arteries

Coronary arteries supply blood to heart tissue. They originate from the aorta.

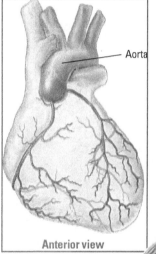

Aorta

Anterior view

Normal coronary artery

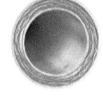

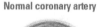
Fatty streak

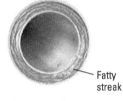
Fibrous plaque

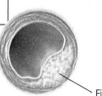
Complicated plaque

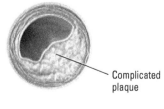

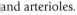

Endocarditis

Endocarditis (also known as *infective* or *bacterial endocarditis*) is an infection of the endocardium, heart valves, or prosthetic heart valves resulting from bacterial or fungal invasion.

How it happens

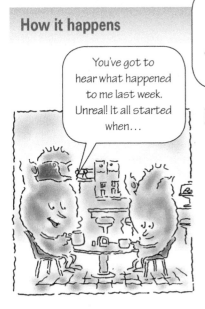

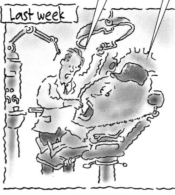

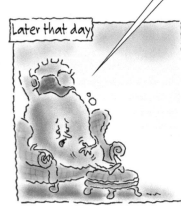

What to look for

- Malaise
- Weakness
- Fatigue
- Weight loss
- Anorexia
- Arthralgia
- Night sweats
- Chills
- Valvular insufficiency (heart murmur)
- Intermittent fever that may recur for weeks (in 90% of patients)

Bacterial endocarditis

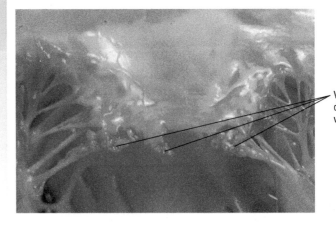

Vegetation destroying valve leaflets

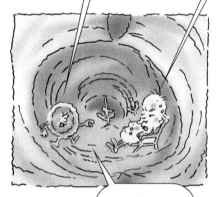

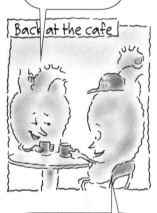

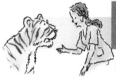

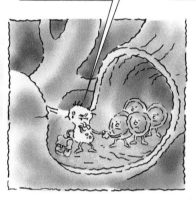

risky business

Risk factors for endocarditis

- Dental procedures
- Immunodeficiency
- I.V. drug use
- Surgery
- Tooth extractions
- Venous access devices, such as central or peripheral catheters
- Artificial heart valves
- Cardiac transplant

Heart failure

Heart failure is a syndrome that occurs when there is a structural or functional impairment of ventricular filling or the heart can't pump enough blood to meet the body's metabolic needs, resulting in intravascular and interstitial volume overload and poor tissue perfusion. Heart failure may be classified as right-sided or left-sided.

How it happens

To the left!

Grab your sidewalk chalk and let's hop around these two pages to learn about heart failure!

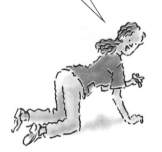

Start

5 The right ventricle may now become stressed because it's pumping against greater pulmonary vascular resistance.
• You may note worsening symptoms.

4 Because the left ventricle can't push all blood volume forward into the aorta, pressure builds up in the left atrium, pulmonary veins, and pulmonary capillaries. High hydrostatic pressure in the pulmonary circulation causes worsening pulmonary edema.
• You may note decreased breath sounds, dullness on percussion, crackles, and orthopnea.

3 Rising capillary pressure pushes sodium (Na) and water (H_2O) into the interstitial space, causing pulmonary edema.
• You may note coughing, crackles, tachypnea, elevated pulmonary capillary wedge pressure, and decreased oxygen saturation of blood.

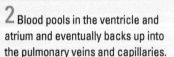

2 Blood pools in the ventricle and atrium and eventually backs up into the pulmonary veins and capillaries.
• You may note dyspnea on exertion, orthopnea, confusion, dizziness, orthostatic hypotension, decreased peripheral pulses and pulse pressure, cyanosis, and an S_3 gallop.

1 Weak heart muscle cannot push total blood volume forward into the aorta; blood accumulates in the left ventricle. Increased workload and end-diastolic volume enlarge the left ventricle.
• You may note increased heart rate, pale and cool skin, tingling in the extremities, decreased cardiac output, and arrhythmias.

6 The stressed right ventricle enlarges with the formation of stretched tissue.
• You may note increased heart rate, cool skin, cyanosis, decreased cardiac output, dyspnea, and palpitations.

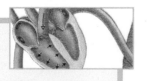

7 Blood pools in the right ventricle and right atrium. The backed-up blood causes pressure and congestion in the vena cava and venous circulation.
• You may note increased central venous pressure, jugular vein distention, and hepatojugular reflux.

To the right!

8 Backed-up blood distends the visceral veins, especially the hepatic and splenic veins. As the liver and spleen become engorged, their function is impaired.
• You may note anorexia, nausea, abdominal pain, palpable liver and spleen, weakness, and dyspnea secondary to abdominal distention (called ascites).

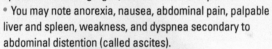

9 Rising capillary pressure forces excess fluid from the capillaries into the interstitial space.
• You may note ankle edema, ascites, weight gain due to excess fluid, and nocturia.

Finish

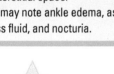

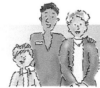

age-old story

Heart failure in children

In children, heart failure occurs mainly as a result of congenital heart defects. Therefore, treatment guidelines are directed toward the specific cause.

Hyperlipidemia

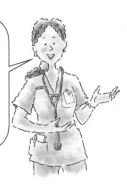

Lipoproteins act as "fat shuttles," transporting cholesterol through the bloodstream.

Hyperlipidemia, also called *lipid disorder*, can be primary or secondary and occurs when there are excess levels of cholesterol and triglycerides. There are mainly two significant types of cholesterol: low-density lipoprotein (LDL), also called "bad cholesterol," and high-density lipoprotein (HDL), also called "good cholesterol."

How it happens

Primary
1 • Inherited autosomal recessive or dominant trait; genetic disorder called familial hypercholesterol-emia

Secondary
2 • Diabetes mellitus
• Pancreatitis
• Hypothyroidism
• Renal disease
• High saturated fat diet
• Habitual excessive alcohol use
• Obesity
• Lack of exercise

What to look for

• Hyperlipidemia most commonly has no symptoms; however, skin deposits of cholesterol are possible.
• Xanthomas (cholesterol deposits under the skin)
• Xanthelasma (cholesterol deposits around the eyes)

A closer look

Cholesterol transport in the blood

Low-density lipoprotein (LDL) travels through the bloodstream and attaches to the lining of the arteries, forming atherosclerotic plaque. High-density lipoprotein (HDL) brings cholesterol to the liver to be excreted as a constituent of bile.

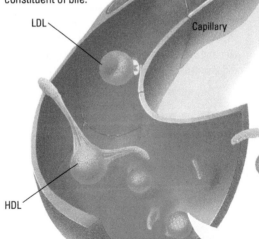

RBCs

LDL

Capillary

HDL

How high cholesterol accumulates in the blood

The liver manufactures cholesterol, and a diet rich in fats causes cholesterol accumulation in blood.

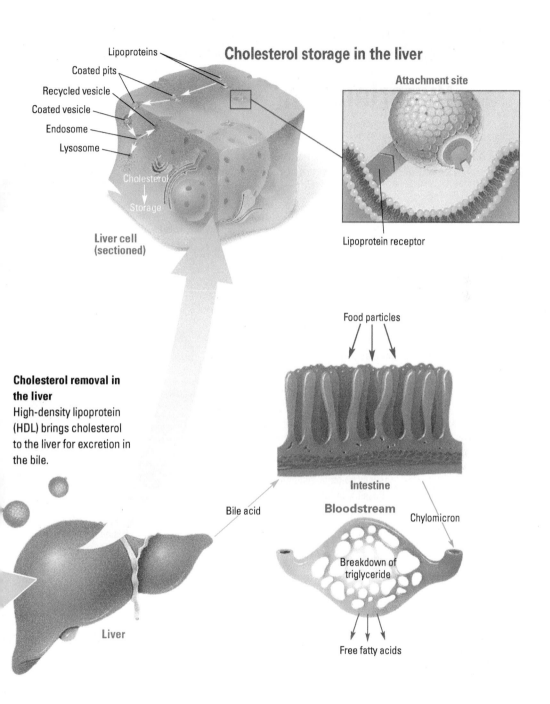

Cholesterol storage in the liver

Lipoproteins

Coated pits

Recycled vesicle

Coated vesicle

Endosome

Lysosome

Cholesterol

Storage

**Liver cell
(sectioned)**

Attachment site

Lipoprotein receptor

**Cholesterol removal in
the liver**
High-density lipoprotein
(HDL) brings cholesterol
to the liver for excretion in
the bile.

Food particles

Intestine

Bloodstream

Bile acid

Chylomicron

Breakdown of
triglyceride

Free fatty acids

Liver

Hypertension

Hypertension is intermittent or sustained elevation of systolic blood pressure greater than 139 mm Hg or diastolic blood pressure greater than 89 mm Hg. Hypertension occurs as essential (primary) hypertension or as secondary hypertension.

How it happens

Several theories exist.

1 Changes in the arteriolar bed cause increased total peripheral resistance (TPR).

2 Abnormally increased tone in the sympathetic nervous system causes increased TPR.

3 Increased arteriolar thickening caused by genetic factors leads to increased TPR.

4 Abnormal renin release results in formation of angiotensin II, which constricts the arterioles and increases blood volume.

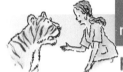

Risk factors for primary hypertension

- Diabetes mellitus
- Family history
- Advancing age
- Obesity
- Sedentary lifestyle
- Stress
- Smoking
- High intake of sodium, saturated fats, and alcohol

What to look for

- Elevated blood pressure (usually no other symptoms)
- Possibly bruits over the abdominal aorta, carotid, renal, and femoral arteries

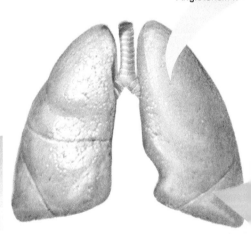

Angiotensin II

3 Angiotensin I is converted to angiotensin II (a potent vasoconstrictor) in the lungs.

Age and systolic hypertension

Elderly people may have isolated systolic hypertension, in which just the systolic blood pressure is elevated, because atherosclerosis causes a loss of elasticity in large arteries.

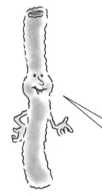

As you get older, you lose elasticity—in your face and in your arteries!

Understanding hypertension

Aldosterone

5 Aldosterone causes sodium and water retention.

1 Kidneys release renin into the bloodstream.

Renin

6 Retained sodium and water increase blood volume.

Aldosterone

4 Angiotensin II causes widespread arteriolar vaso-constriction in the body and stimulates adrenal gland to release aldosterone.

2 Renin stimulates angio-tensinogen formation in the liver. Angiotensinogen becomes angiotensin I.

Angiotensin

Angiotensin I

8 Increased blood volume and vascular resistance cause hypertension.

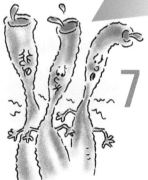

7 Arteriolar constriction increases peripheral vascular resistance.

Hypovolemic shock

In hypovolemic shock, reduced intravascular volume causes lack of circulation and inadequate tissue perfusion. It's commonly caused by acute blood loss— about 20% of total volume—that can result from:

- Bleeding, internal or external hemorrhage, or a condition that reduces circulating intravascular volume or levels of other fluids
- Traumatic injury that causes bleeding
- Obstetrical complications, such as abruptio placenta or placenta previa, which cause bleeding
- Burns
- Dehydration from excessive perspiration, severe diarrhea, protracted vomiting, diabetes insipidus, diuresis, or inadequate fluid intake
- Third-space fluid shift, which can occur in the abdominal cavity (ascites), pleural cavity, or pericardial sac, can also cause hypovolemic shock.

How it happens

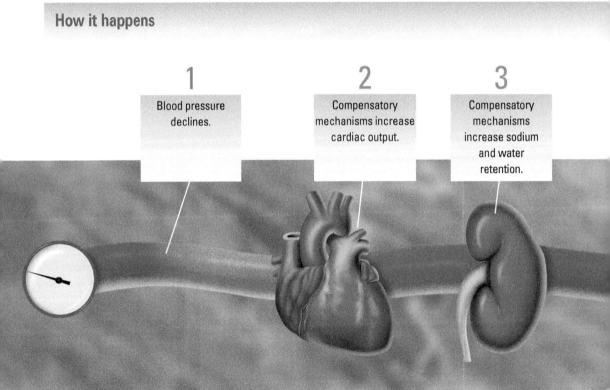

1
Blood pressure declines.

2
Compensatory mechanisms increase cardiac output.

3
Compensatory mechanisms increase sodium and water retention.

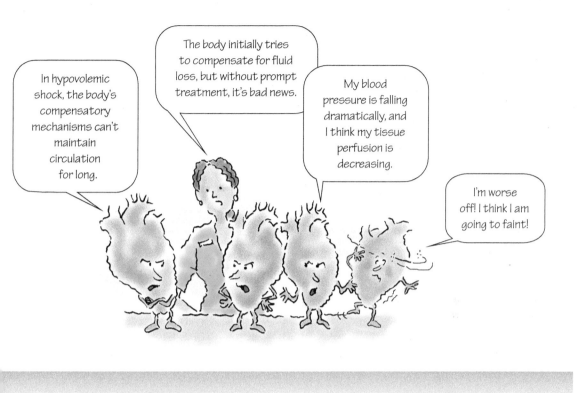

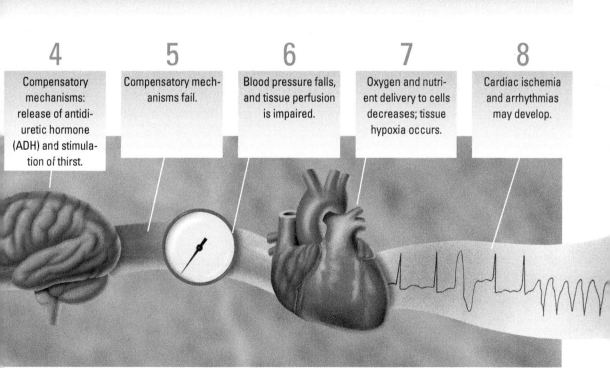

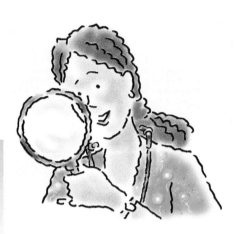

What to look for

* Severe hypotension
* Cool, clammy skin
* Weak, thready pulse
* Pallor
* Dizziness
* Syncope (fainting)
* Decreased urine output

INCREASED

* Heart rate
* Respirations
* Serum creatinine and blood urea nitrogen (BUN) levels

DECREASED

* Cardiac output (CO)
* Sensorium
* Pulse pressure
* Urine output (<25 mL/hour)
* Blood pressure
* Central venous pressure, pulmonary artery pressure, and pulmonary capillary wedge pressure
* Hemoglobin (Hgb) level
* Hematocrit (Hct)

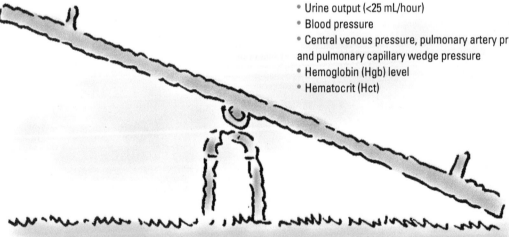

Myocarditis

Myocarditis is focal or diffuse inflammation of the cardiac muscle (myocardium). It may be acute or chronic and can occur at any age.

How it happens

Damage to the myocardium occurs when an infectious organism (commonly a virus) triggers an autoimmune reaction. The resulting inflammation may lead to hypertrophy, fibrosis, and inflammatory changes of the myocardium and conduction system. The heart muscle weakens, and contractility is reduced. The heart muscle becomes flabby and dilated.

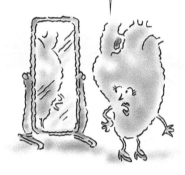

Honestly, does this look flabby to you?

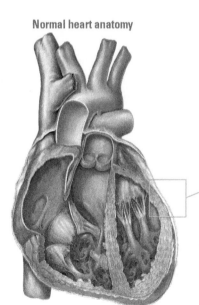

Normal heart anatomy

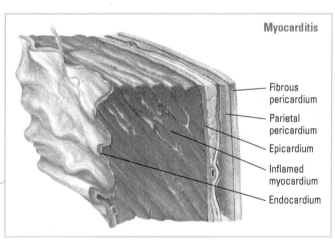

Myocarditis

- Fibrous pericardium
- Parietal pericardium
- Epicardium
- Inflamed myocardium
- Endocardium

What to look for

- Fatigue
- Dyspnea
- Palpitations
- Fever
- Mild, continuous pressure or soreness in the chest
- Tachycardia
- S_3 and S_4 gallops
- Peripheral edema

Pericarditis

Pericarditis is an inflammation of the pericardium. Acute pericarditis can be fibrinous or effusive, with purulent, serous, or hemorrhagic exudate. Chronic constrictive pericarditis is characterized by dense, fibrous pericardial thickening.

How it happens

- Bacterial, fungal, or viral infection
- Neoplasms
- High-dose radiation to the chest
- Autoimmune disease such as systemic lupus erythematosus
- Drugs, such as hydralazine or procainamide
- Infection after cardiac surgery
- Post–myocardial infarction inflammation

The inflammatory process in pericarditis

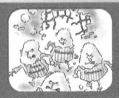 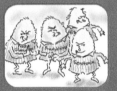 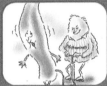 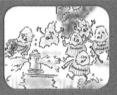 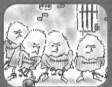

1 Pericardial tissue damaged by bacteria or other substances releases chemical mediators of inflammation into the surrounding tissue.

2 Friction occurs as the inflamed pericardial layers rub against each other.

3 Histamines and other chemical mediators dilate vessels and increase vessel permeability.

4 Fluids and protein (including fibrinogen) leak into the tissues, causing extracellular edema. Macrophages, neutrophils, and monocytes in the tissue begin to phagocytose the invading bacteria.

5 Gradually, the space fills with an exudate composed of necrotic tissue, dead and dying bacteria, neutrophils, and macrophages. These products are eventually reabsorbed into healthy tissue.

What to look for

- Pericardial friction rub
- Sharp, sudden pain starting at the sternum and radiating to the neck, shoulders, and arms
- Shallow, rapid respirations
- Mild fever
- Dyspnea
- Orthopnea
- Tachycardia
- Muffled and distant heart sounds
- Fluid retention
- Ascites
- Hepatomegaly
- Jugular vein distention

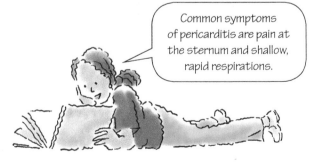

Common symptoms of pericarditis are pain at the sternum and shallow, rapid respirations.

Valvular heart disease

Aortic insufficiency

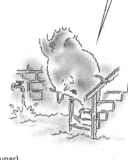

Uh oh...I think someone forgot to shut off the aortic valve!

Aortic insufficiency is the incomplete closure of the aortic valve. It can be acute or chronic and is usually caused by scarring or retraction of valve leaflets.

In aortic insufficiency, blood flows back into the left ventricle during diastole, causing fluid overload in the ventricle, which dilates and hypertrophies. The backup and leakage is referred to as aortic regurgitation. The excess volume causes fluid overload backward into the left atrium and pulmonary veins and, finally, into the pulmonary capillaries. Left-sided heart failure and pulmonary edema eventually result.

How it happens

Acute
- Endocarditis
- Chest trauma
- Prosthetic valve malfunction
- Acute ascending aortic dissection

Chronic
- Hypertension
- Rheumatic fever
- Marfan syndrome
- Ankylosing spondylitis
- Syphilis
- Ventricular septal defect

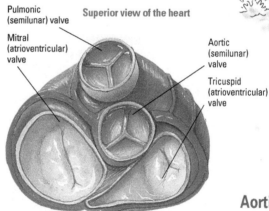

Superior view of the heart

Pulmonic (semilunar) valve

Mitral (atrioventricular) valve

Aortic (semilunar) valve

Tricuspid (atrioventricular) valve

What to look for

- Pulmonary crackles
- Shock
- Dyspnea
- Orthopnea
- Paroxysmal nocturnal dyspnea
- Fatigue
- Exercise intolerance
- S_3 heart sound
- Angina
- Palpitations
- Widened pulse pressure
- Diastolic blowing murmur at the left sternal border

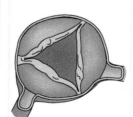

Retracted fibrosed valve leaflets

Aortic insufficiency

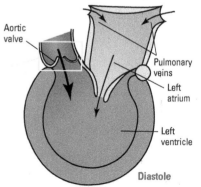

Aortic valve

Pulmonary veins

Left atrium

Left ventricle

Diastole

Valvular heart disease

Aortic stenosis

Aortic stenosis is a narrowing of the aortic valve. Aortic valve narrowing hinders blood flow into the aorta decreasing arterial circulation and coronary circulation. A narrow aortic valve also increases the resistance against the left ventricle making the left ventricle hypertrophy. An enlarged left ventricular muscle requires greater coronary blood flow, which is not available. Thus, ischemia of the left ventricle occurs causing angina and eventually heart failure.

How it happens

Aortic stenosis can occur as a result of the following:
- Aortic valve calcification due to aging
- Congenital aortic bicuspid valve
- Rheumatic fever
- Atherosclerosis

What to look for

- Loud systolic murmur
- Angina
- Syncope
- Dyspnea

Aortic valve stenosis

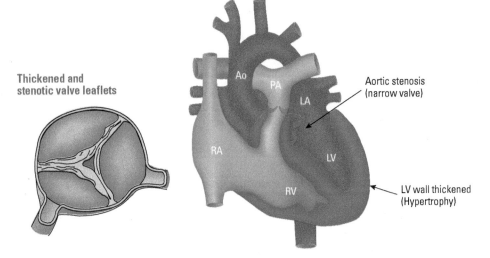

Thickened and stenotic valve leaflets

Ao

PA

LA

RA

LV

RV

Aortic stenosis (narrow valve)

LV wall thickened (Hypertrophy)

Valvular heart disease

Mitral insufficiency

An abnormality of the mitral leaflets, mitral annulus, chordae tendineae, papillary muscles, left atrium, or left ventricle can lead to mitral insufficiency, also called mitral regurgitation. Mitral insufficiency causes leakage of blood into the left atrium during systole through a loose mitral valve. Blood volume increases in the left atrium, backward into the pulmonary veins and pulmonary capillaries. With high volume in the pulmonary capillaries, pulmonary edema results. Also, the left atrium will dilate due to backflow of blood. An enlarged left atrium can lead to atrial fibrillation.

There's too much flowing from the left ventricle into the left atrium. I can't accommodate all of this backflow!

How it happens

Mitral insufficiency can occur as a result of the following:
* Rheumatic fever
* Mitral valve prolapse
* Hypertrophic obstructive cardiomyopathy
* Myocardial infarction
* Ruptured chordae tendineae

What to look for

* Pulmonary edema (crackles)
* Exertional dyspnea
* Paroxysmal nocturnal dyspnea
* Orthopnea
* Weakness
* Fatigue
* Palpitations
* Atrial fibrillation
* Irregular pulse
* An opening snap and a holosystolic murmur at the apex

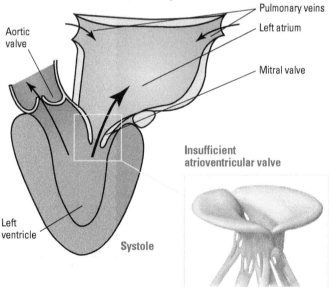

Mitral valve insufficiency

Pulmonary veins

Left atrium

Mitral valve

Aortic valve

Left ventricle

Systole

Insufficient atrioventricular valve

Valvular heart disease

Mitral prolapse

Mitral valve prolapse is a billowing and subsequent improper closing of the mitral valve that causes mitral regurgitation, backflow of blood into the left atrium. The left atrium becomes overloaded and dilates, which can lead to atrial fibrillation. There are episodes of low blood flow into the left ventricle from the left atrium and decreased blood flow into the aorta. With decreased blood flow into the aorta, the coronary arteries sustain decreased blood flow, which can cause episodes of coronary insufficiency leading to chest pain and syncope. It is episodic and occurs more frequently in women than in men.

memory board

In valvular heart disease, the heart's mitral valve can be subjected to three types of disruption. To help you remember them, just think **SIP**:

Stenosis

Insufficiency

Prolapse.

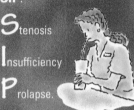

What to look for

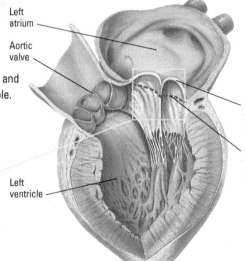

Dizziness, syncope, palpitations, chest pain, and heart murmur? Just as I suspected—mitral prolapse, I presume.

How it happens

Mitral valve prolapse can occur as a result of the following:
- Autosomal dominant inheritance
- Genetic or environmental interruption of valve development during gestation
- Inherited connective tissue disorders, such as Ehlers-Danlos syndrome, Marfan syndrome, and osteogenesis imperfecta

Mitral valve prolapse

A view of the mitral valve from the left atrium shows redundant and deformed leaflets that billow up into the left atrium during systole.

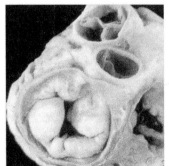

Cross section of left ventricle

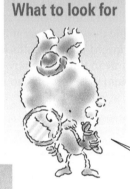

Left atrium

Aortic valve

Left ventricle

Prolapse valve (closed)

Normal valve (closed)

Valvular heart disease

Mitral stenosis

How it happens

Mitral stenosis can occur as a result of the following:
- Rheumatic fever
- Congenital abnormalities
- Atrial myxoma
- Calcification of the mitral valve in elderly population
- Endocarditis

Mitral valve stenosis

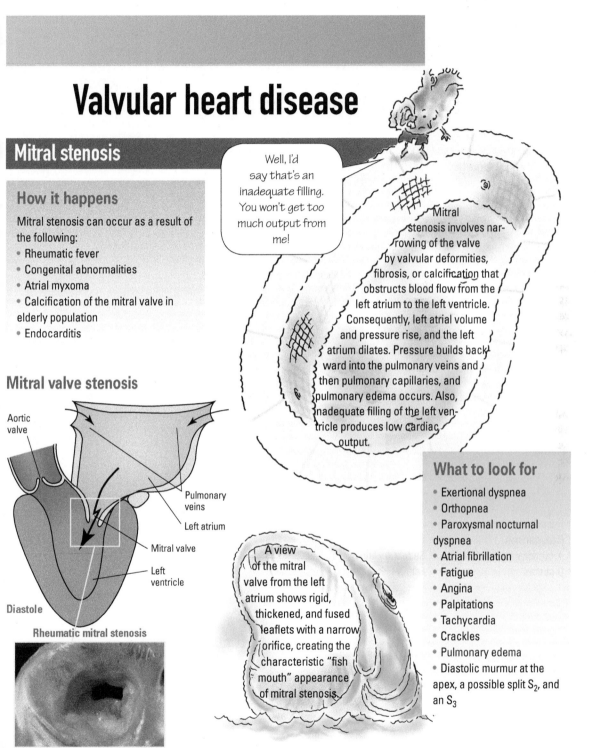

Well, I'd say that's an inadequate filling. You won't get too much output from me!

Mitral stenosis involves narrowing of the valve by valvular deformities, fibrosis, or calcification that obstructs blood flow from the left atrium to the left ventricle. Consequently, left atrial volume and pressure rise, and the left atrium dilates. Pressure builds backward into the pulmonary veins and then pulmonary capillaries, and pulmonary edema occurs. Also, inadequate filling of the left ventricle produces low cardiac output.

Aortic valve

Pulmonary veins

Left atrium

Mitral valve

Left ventricle

Diastole

Rheumatic mitral stenosis

A view of the mitral valve from the left atrium shows rigid, thickened, and fused leaflets with a narrow orifice, creating the characteristic "fish mouth" appearance of mitral stenosis.

What to look for
- Exertional dyspnea
- Orthopnea
- Paroxysmal nocturnal dyspnea
- Atrial fibrillation
- Fatigue
- Angina
- Palpitations
- Tachycardia
- Crackles
- Pulmonary edema
- Diastolic murmur at the apex, a possible split S_2, and an S_3

Peripheral arterial disease

Peripheral arterial disease (PAD), also called arterial insufficiency, is a disease caused by arteriosclerosis of the lower extremity. There is arteriosclerotic plaque obstructing arterial blood flow into the leg. The leg muscle can become ischemic or infarcted if not treated.

How it happens

The lining of an artery in the leg accumulates arteriosclerotic plaque. The plaque becomes large enough to hinder arterial blood flow into the leg. This is most evident during physical activity when the muscle requires greater circulation. The lack of sufficient arterial blood flow causes ischemia and symptoms in the leg.

What to look for

* Pain in the leg with activity (called intermittent claudication)
* Paresthesias (numbness and tingling in the foot)
* Palpable coolness of the leg
* Paresis (weakness) or paralysis of the leg
* Pulselessness in the leg

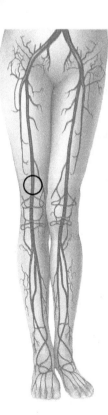

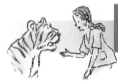

risky business

Risk Factors

* Hyperlipidemia
* Hypertension
* Arteriosclerosis
* Diabetes

* Coronary artery disease
* Smoking
* Sedentary lifestyle
* Family history

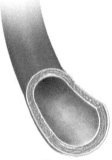

Normal Artery

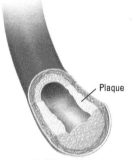

Plaque

Build up of fatty substances in the wall of the artery

Deep vein thrombosis

Deep vein thrombosis (DVT), also called venous thromboembolism, is a disorder that involves inflammation and clot formation in a deep vein of the leg. The venous clot can travel from the leg into the inferior vena cava and then into the right side of the heart. From the right ventricle, the clot can travel into the pulmonary artery and the lungs. When in the lungs, the clot, called a pulmonary embolism (PE) at that stage, can obstruct circulation in the lung and hinder oxygen transfer from alveoli into the blood. A large PE can be fatal.

risky business

Risk Factors

There are three risk factors for DVT, called Virchow triad:
1—Venous stasis
2—Vein injury
3—Hypercoagulability of the blood

How it happens

DVT occurs most often due to venous pooling of the blood in the lower extremities. Often, this is due to a sedentary position of the leg for a prolonged amount of time. When venous blood is stagnant, it is susceptible to clot formation. A clot then forms in the leg and travels up to the lungs and becomes a pulmonary embolism. DVT also occurs in disorders where the blood is hypercoagulable such as pregnancy or cancer. Orthopedic surgery is a major risk factor for DVT because the patient is subjected to vein injury during surgery and then is on bed rest in the recovery period, which causes stasis of venous blood.

What to look for in PE

- Sudden dyspnea
- Chest pain
- Tachycardia
- However, PE is most often without symptoms.

What to look for in DVT

- Redness over a vein
- Warmth over a vein
- Tenderness over a vein
- Ropiness over a vein
- Edema of the leg
- However, most often, DVT occurs without symptoms.

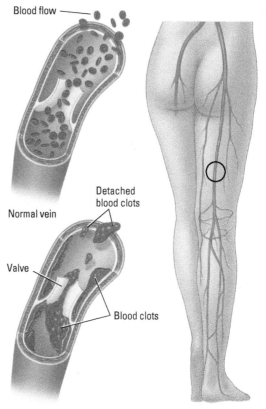

Blood flow

Normal vein

Valve

Detached blood clots

Blood clots

DVT

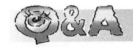

Matchmaker

Match the definitions given here with their corresponding disorders.

1. Inflammation of the pericardium _____

2. An infection of the endocardium, heart valves, or cardiac prosthesis _____

3. An abnormal dilation in the aortic arterial wall _____

4. An unchecked increase in pressure in the pericardial sac _____

5. Narrowing of the aortic valve _____

6. A disease of heart muscle fibers _____

A. Cardiomyopathy

B. Aortic stenosis

C. Cardiac tamponade

D. Endocarditis

E. Aortic aneurysm

F. Pericarditis

Riddle

Solve the riddle to find an important fact about coronary artery disease.

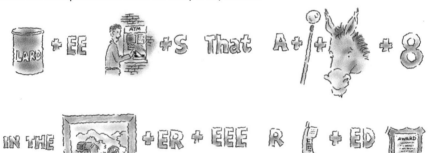

Selected References

American Heart Association. (2015). Types of heart failure. Retrieved from http://www.heart.org/HEARTORG/Conditions/HeartFailure/AboutHeartFailure/Types-of-Heart-Failure_UCM_306323_Article.jsp on May 2015.

Amsterdam, E. A., Wenger, N. K., Brindisi, R. G., Casey, D. E., Jr., Ganiats, T. G., Holmes, D. R., Jr., …, Zieman, S. J. (2014). AHA/ACC guideline for the management of patients with non–ST-elevation acute coronary syndromes: A report of the American College of Cardiology/American Heart Association Task Force on Practice Guidelines. *Journal of the American College of Cardiology, 64*(24), e139–228.

Anderson, M. W., & Watson, G. A. (2013). Traumatic shock: The fifth shock. *Journal of Trauma Nursing, 20*(1), 37–43.

Bodson, L., Bouferrache, K., & Vieillard-Baron, A. (2011). Cardiac tamponade. *Current Opinion in Critical Care, 17*(5), 416–424.

Cannon, C. P., Brindis, R. G., Chaitman, B. R., Cohen, D. J., Cross, J. T., Jr., Drozda, J. P., Jr., …, Weintraub, W. S. (2013). ACCF/AHA key data elements and definitions for measuring the clinical management and outcomes of patients with acute coronary syndromes and coronary artery disease: A report of the American College of Cardiology Foundation/American Heart Association Task Force on Clinical Data Standards (Writing Committee to Develop Acute Coronary Syndromes and Coronary Artery Disease Clinical Data Standards). *Journal of the American College of Cardiology, 61*(9), 992–1025.

Curry, S. (2014). Acute pericarditis: An overview. *British Journal of Cardiac Nursing, 9*(3), 124–131.

Elamm, C., Fairweather, D., & Cooper, L. T. (2012). Pathogenesis and diagnosis of myocarditis. *Heart, 98*(11), 835–840.

Gersh, B. J., Maron, B. J., Bonow, R. O., Dearani, J. A., Fifer, M. A., Link, M. S., …, Yancy, C. W. (2011). ACCF/AHA guideline for the diagnosis and treatment of hypertrophic cardiomyopathy: A report of the American College of Cardiology Foundation/American Heart Association Task Force on Practice Guidelines. *Circulation, 124*(24), e783–e831.

Kumar, V., Abbas, A., & Aster, J. (2015). *Robbins & Cotran pathologic basis of disease*. Philadelphia, PA: Elsevier, Saunders.

Linden, B. (2015). Recommendations for care of patients with acute coronary syndromes. *British Journal of Cardiac Nursing, 10*(1), 8–9.

Miller, M., Stone, N. J., Ballantyne, C., Bittner, V., Criqui, M. H., Ginsberg, H. N., …, Pennathur, S.; on behalf of the American Heart Association Clinical Lipidology, Thrombosis, and Prevention Committee of the Council on Nutrition, Physical Activity and Metabolism, Council on Arteriosclerosis, Thrombosis and Vascular Biology, Council on Cardiovascular Nursing, and Council on the Kidney in Cardiovascular Disease. (2011). Triglycerides and cardiovascular disease: A scientific statement from the American Heart Association. *Circulation, 123*(20), 2292–2333.

Nishimura, R. A., Otto, C. M., Bonow, R. O., Carabello, B. A., Erwin, J. P., III, Guyton, R. A., …, Thomas, J. D. (2014). AHA/ACC guideline for the management of patients with valvular heart disease: Executive summary: a report of the American College of Cardiology/American Heart Association Task Force on Practice Guidelines. *Circulation, 129*(23), e650.

O'Donovan, K. (2011). Cardiogenic shock complicating myocardial infarction: An overview. *British Journal of Cardiac Nursing, 6*(6), 280–285.

Riley, J. (2013). Acute decompensated heart failure: Diagnosis and management. *British Journal of Nursing, 22*(22), 1290–1295.

Rosendorff, C., Lackland, D. T., Allison, M., Aronow, W. S., Black, H. R., Blumenthal, R. S., …, White, W. B.; on behalf of the American Heart Association, American College of Cardiology, and American Society of Hypertension. (2015). Treatment of hypertension in patients with coronary artery disease: A scientific statement from the American Heart Association, American College of Cardiology, and American Society of Hypertension. *Circulation, 131*(19), e435–e470.

Smith, S. C., Jr, Benjamin, E. J., Bonow, R. O., Braun, L. T., Creager, M. A., Franklin, B. A., …, Taubert, K. A. (2011). AHA/ACCF secondary prevention and risk reduction therapy for patients with coronary and other atherosclerotic vascular disease: 2011 Update: A guideline from the American Heart Association and American College of Cardiology Foundation. *Circulation, 124*(22), 2458–2473.

White, A., & Broder, J. (2012). Acute aortic emergencies—Part 1: Aortic aneurysms. *Emergency Nursing Journal, 34*(3), 216–229.

Yancy, C. W., Jessup, M., Bozkurt, B., Butler, J., Casey, D. E., Jr, Drazner, M. H., …, Wilkoff, B. L. (2013). ACCF/AHA guideline for the management of heart failure: A report of the American College of Cardiology Foundation/American Heart Association Task Force on Practice Guidelines. *Circulation, 128*(16), e240–e327.

Chapter 3

Respiratory disorders

 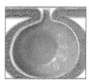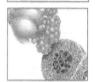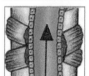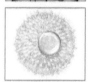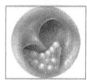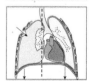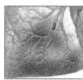
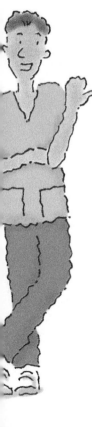

Acute respiratory distress syndrome

Respiratory

Acute respiratory distress syndrome (ARDS) is a form of pulmonary edema that can quickly lead to acute respiratory failure. Also known as *shock lung,* ARDS may follow a direct or indirect lung injury. It's difficult to diagnose and can prove fatal within 48 hours of onset if not promptly diagnosed and treated. Mortality associated with ARDS remains at 50% to 70%. Many people who do recover suffer long-term lung damage and oxygen deprivation during the illness.

A closer look

Phase 2

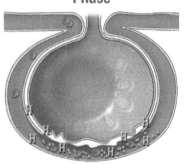

In *phase 2,* those substances—especially histamine—inflame and damage the alveolar-capillary membrane, increasing capillary permeability. Fluids then shift into the interstitial space.

Phase 1

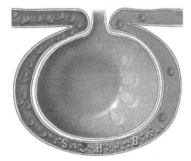

In *phase 1,* injury reduces normal blood flow to the lungs. Platelets aggregate and release histamine (H), serotonin (S), and bradykinin (B).

How it happens

Shock, sepsis, and trauma are the most common causes of ARDS. Trauma-related factors, such as fat emboli, pulmonary contusions, and multiple transfusions, may increase the likelihood that microemboli will develop.

3

Phase

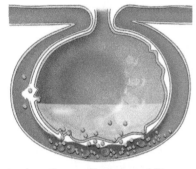

In *phase 3,* as capillary permeability increases, proteins and fluids leak out, increasing interstitial osmotic pressure and causing pulmonary edema.

4

Phase

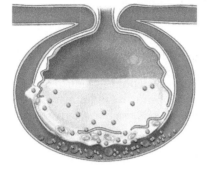

In *phase 4,* decreased blood flow and fluids in the alveoli damage surfactant and impair the cell's ability to produce more. As a result, alveoli collapse, impeding gas exchange and decreasing lung compliance.

What to look for

- Rapid, shallow breathing
- Dyspnea
- Hypoxemia
- Intercostal and suprasternal retractions
- Crackles
- Rhonchi
- Restlessness
- Apprehension
- Decreased level of consciousness
- Tachycardia

Severe ARDS

- Hypotension
- Decreased urine output
- Respiratory and metabolic acidosis
- Diminished ability to breathe independently
- Loss of consciousness, coma

5

Phase

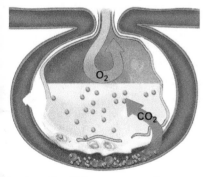

In *phase 5,* sufficient oxygen can't cross the alveolar-capillary membrane, but carbon dioxide (CO_2) can and is lost with every exhalation. Oxygen (O_2) and CO_2 levels decrease in the blood.

6

Phase

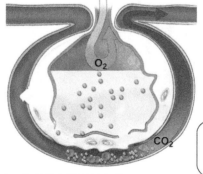

In *phase 6,* pulmonary edema worsens, inflammation leads to fibrosis, and gas exchange is further impeded.

memory board

Antibiotics

Respiratory support

Diuretics

Situate the patient in the prone position

Use the abbreviation for ARDS to remember key treatments.

Asthma

Asthma is a chronic reactive airway disorder that can present as an acute attack. It causes episodic airway obstruction resulting from bronchospasms, increased mucus secretion, and mucosal edema. Asthma is one type of chronic obstructive pulmonary disease (COPD), a long-term pulmonary disease characterized by airflow resistance.

Cases of asthma continue to rise. It currently affects an estimated 17 million Americans; children account for 4.8 million asthma sufferers in the United States.

A case of exposure

1st exposure

1 Allergens may enter through the nose and mouth.

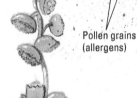

Ragweed

Pollen grains (allergens)

How it happens

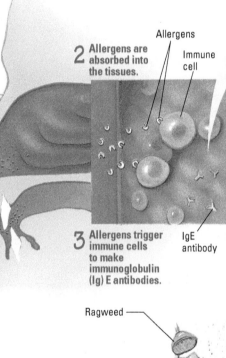

2 Allergens are absorbed into the tissues.

Allergens

Immune cell

3 Allergens trigger immune cells to make immunoglobulin (Ig) E antibodies.

IgE antibody

Ragweed

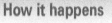

age-old story

Age and asthma

Although asthma strikes at any age, about 50% of patients are younger than age 10; twice as many boys as girls are affected in this age-group. One-third of patients develop asthma from ages 10 to 30, and the incidence is the same in both sexes in this age-group. African Americans and those living in poverty are at higher risk of developing asthma.

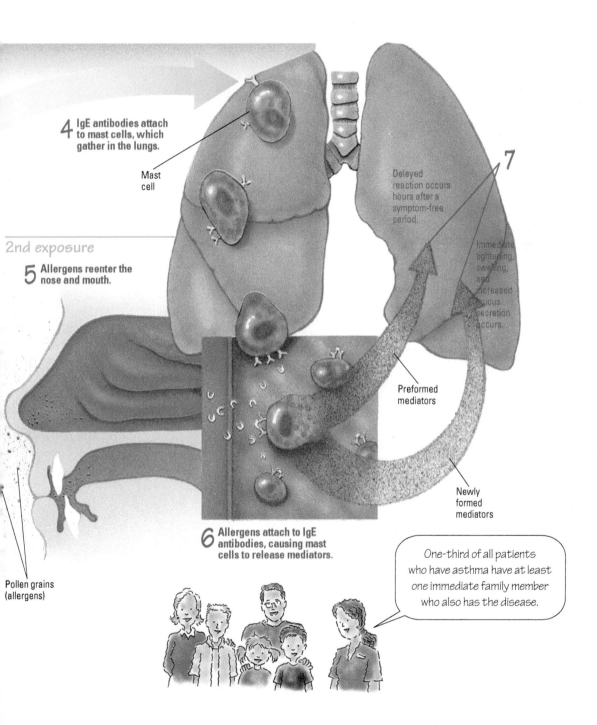

4 IgE antibodies attach to mast cells, which gather in the lungs.

Mast cell

2nd exposure

5 Allergens reenter the nose and mouth.

Delayed reaction occurs hours after a symptom-free period.

Immediate tightening, swelling, and increased mucus secretion occurs.

7

Preformed mediators

Newly formed mediators

6 Allergens attach to IgE antibodies, causing mast cells to release mediators.

Pollen grains (allergens)

One-third of all patients who have asthma have at least one immediate family member who also has the disease.

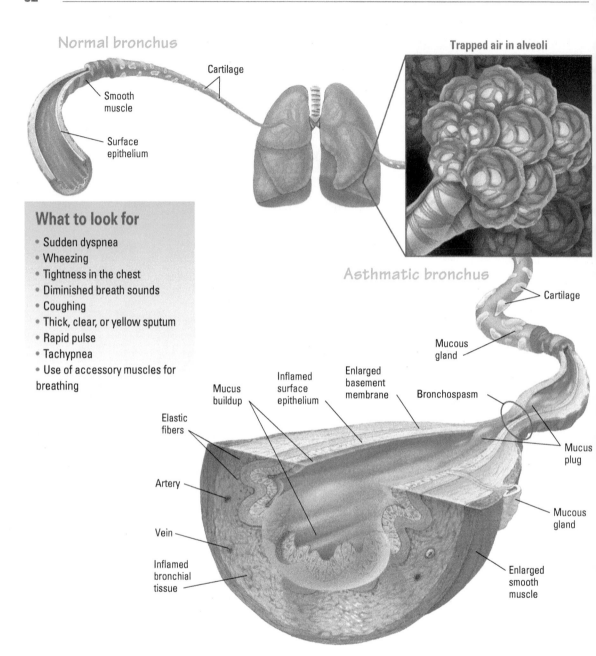

Normal bronchus

Cartilage

Smooth muscle

Surface epithelium

Trapped air in alveoli

What to look for

- Sudden dyspnea
- Wheezing
- Tightness in the chest
- Diminished breath sounds
- Coughing
- Thick, clear, or yellow sputum
- Rapid pulse
- Tachypnea
- Use of accessory muscles for breathing

Asthmatic bronchus

Cartilage

Mucous gland

Bronchospasm

Inflamed surface epithelium

Enlarged basement membrane

Mucus buildup

Mucus plug

Elastic fibers

Artery

Vein

Inflamed bronchial tissue

Mucous gland

Enlarged smooth muscle

Chronic bronchitis

Chronic bronchitis, a form of COPD, is inflammation of the bronchi caused by irritants or infection.

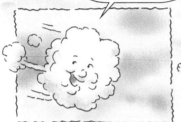

My job as airflow is vital to breathing!

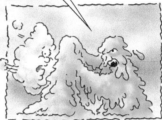

This is my second straight year of hanging around longer than 3 months. I love being a menace!

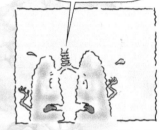

That mucus is blocking my airflow! Chronic bronchitis can't be far behind!

How it happens

Chronic bronchitis causes inflammation and mucous accumulation in the airways which narrows the bronchioles and leads to decreased oxygen entering alveoli and hypoxia.

Chronic hypoxia eventually causes pulmonary arteriole vasoconstriction leading to high pressure in the pulmonary system; also known as pulmonary hypertension. As pulmonary pressure rises, the right ventricle has increasing resistance against it and eventually right sided heart failure occurs.

Chronic hypoxia also causes the kidneys to produce erythropoetin which leads to RBC production leading to polycythemia. The Hgb level is high but the amount of oxygen is low, therefore cyanosis is evident.

Healthy bronchi

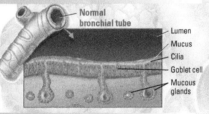

- Normal bronchial tube
- Lumen
- Mucus
- Cilia
- Goblet cell
- Mucous glands

Chronic bronchitis

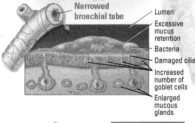

- Narrowed bronchial tube
- Lumen
- Excessive mucus retention
- Bacteria
- Damaged cilia
- Increased number of goblet cells
- Enlarged mucous glands

What to look for

- Productive cough
- Dyspnea
- Cyanosis
- Use of accessory muscles for breathing
- Pulmonary hypertension

age-old story

Age and chronic bronchitis

Children of parents who smoke are at higher risk for respiratory tract infection that can lead to chronic bronchitis.

Cor pulmonale

In cor pulmonale, hypertrophy and dilation of the right ventricle develop secondary to a disease affecting the structure or function of the lungs or associated structures. Lung disease occurs first, leading to consequences for the right side of the heart.

Cor pulmonale occurs at the end stage of various disorders of the lungs that cause chronic hypoxia such as COPD. The chronic hypoxia causes pulmonary arteriole vasoconstriction, which leads to pulmonary hypertension. High pressure in the pulmonary arteriole system leads to high workload for the right ventricle and eventual right ventricular failure.

Cor pulmonale causes about 25% of all types of heart failure. About 85% of patients with cor pulmonale also have COPD, and about 25% of patients with bronchial COPD eventually develop cor pulmonale. It's most common in smokers and middle-aged and elderly men; however, incidence in women is rising.

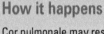

How it happens

Cor pulmonale may result from any disorders that cause chronic hypoxia and resultant pulmonary hypertension such as the following:
- COPD, which includes chronic bronchitis or emphysema
- Bronchopulmonary dysplasia
- Bronchiectasis
- Cystic fibrosis
- Pulmonary fibrosis
- Pulmonary vascular diseases, such as vasculitis or pulmonary emboli
- Pulmonary autoimmune disease

Pulmonary disorder

⬇

Anatomic alterations in the pulmonary blood vessels and functional alterations in the lung

⬇

Increased pulmonary vascular resistance

⬇

Pulmonary hypertension

⬇

Right ventricular hypertrophy (cor pulmonale)

⬇

Heart failure

What to look for

Early
- Chronic, productive cough
- Exertional dyspnea
- Wheezing
- Fatigue and weakness

Progressive
- Dyspnea at rest
- Tachypnea
- Orthopnea
- Dependent edema
- Distended jugular veins
- Hepatomegaly (enlarged, tender liver)
- Hepatojugular reflux (jugular vein distention induced by pressing over the liver)
- Tachycardia
- Decreased cardiac output
- Weight gain due to edema

Cross-section of the heart with cor pulmonale

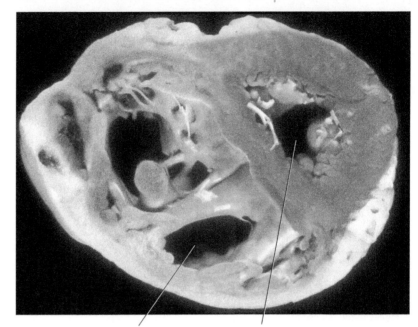

Right ventricle   Left ventricle

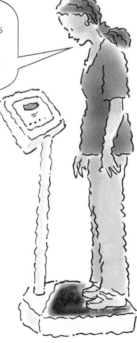

Weight gain due to edema is one of the symptoms of progressive cor pulmonale. Best to keep those lungs and heart healthy!

age-old story

Age and cor pulmonale

In children, cor pulmonale may be a complication of cystic fibrosis, upper airway obstruction, scleroderma, extensive bronchiectasis, or neuromuscular diseases that affect respiratory muscles.

Emphysema

Chronic obstructive pulmonary disease (COPD) consists of chronic bronchitis, emphysema, and asthma. All three diseases are present in COPD. In emphysema, there is abnormal, permanent enlargement of the alveoli due to destruction of the integrity of the alveolar walls. Alveoli become overly distended with air and cannot recoil to release CO_2.

The distinguishing characteristic of emphysema is airflow limitation caused by a lack of elastic recoil in the lungs.

How it happens

In emphysema, recurrent inflammation is associated with the release of proteolytic enzymes (enzymes that promote breakdown) from lung cells. This causes irreversible enlargement of the air spaces distal to the terminal bronchioles. Enlargement of air spaces destroys the alveolar walls, which results in a breakdown of elasticity, making the lungs less compliant.

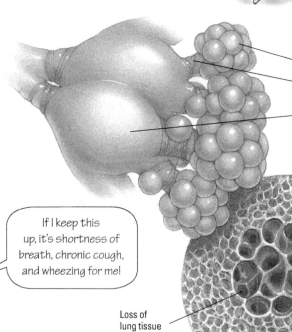

Lung changes in emphysema

- Alveolus
- Smooth muscle
- Dilation and destruction of bronchial walls
- Loss of lung tissue

What to look for

- Tachypnea
- Exertional dyspnea
- Barrel-shaped chest
- Prolonged expiration
- Decreased breath sounds
- Clubbed fingers and toes
- Decreased tactile fremitus
- Decreased chest expansion
- Hyperresonance
- Wheezing on inspiration

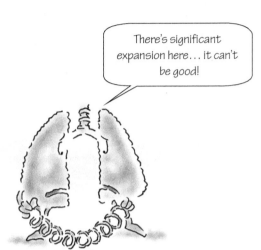

There's significant expansion here... it can't be good!

Air trapping in emphysema

After alveolar walls are damaged or destroyed, they lose their capability of elastic recoil. Air accumulates in the distended alveoli. The person with emphysema develops a barrel-shaped chest due to excess air in the lungs.

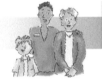

age-old story

Age and emphysema

Aging is a risk factor for emphysema. Senile emphysema results from degenerative changes of the alveoli that occurs with age. The alveolar membranes lose recoiling ability, which causes overdistention of the alveoli.

Normal expiration

Note normal recoil and the open bronchiole.

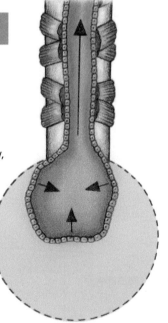

Impaired expiration occurs in COPD

Note decreased elastic recoil (occur in emphysema) and a narrowed bronchiole (occur in chronic bronchitis).

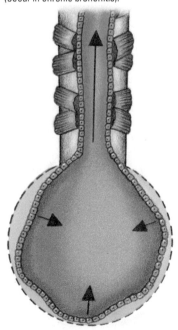

Influenza

Influenza, also known as the *flu* or *grippe*, is an acute, highly contagious viral infection of the respiratory tract. Influenza occurs sporadically or in epidemics (appears as early as October; activity peaks in January). Epidemics usually peak in 2 to 3 weeks after initial cases appear and last 2 to 3 months.

Influenza results from three types of virus.

How it happens

Type A

Type A, the most prevalent, strikes every year, and causes the most severe symptoms.

Type B

Type B also strikes annually causing less severe symptoms.

Type C

Type C causes only sporadic cases.

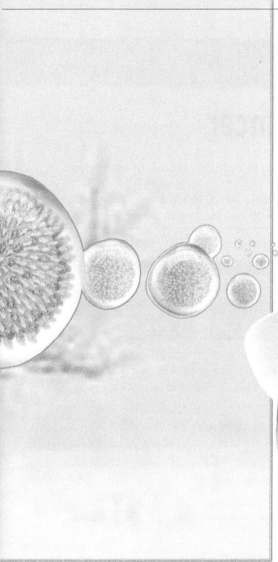

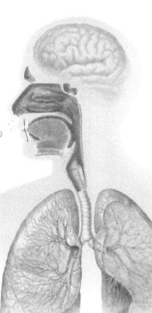

Understanding influenza

Influenza spreads in the droplets that spray out of an infected person's mouth and nose when the person sneezes or coughs, laughs, or even talks. When someone else breathes in these droplets or gets them on his or her hands and then touches his or her own mouth or nose, the virus can enter his or her body. The best way to prevent influenza is the annual vaccine.

What to look for

- Fever
- Chills
- Headache
- Fatigue, weakness
- Runny or stuffy nose
- Sneezing
- Sore throat
- Cough
- Chest discomfort
- General aches and pains
- Bronchitis

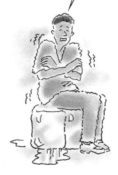

> Fever, headache, sneezing…I'm afraid I must have had an unfortunate meeting with some droplets!

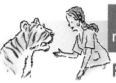

risky business

Risk factors for complications of influenza

- Age 65 and older
- Ages 6 to 23 months
- Any age with chronic medical conditions
- Immunosuppression
- COPD

Lung cancer

Although lung cancer is largely preventable, it remains the most common cause of cancer death in men and women.

About 80% of lung cancers are non-small-cell lung cancer, which includes three subtypes. The cells in these subtypes differ in size, shape, and chemical makeup and are described here.

Adenocarcinoma	Squamous cell	Large-cell undifferentiated
• Usually found in the outer region of the lung	• Commonly linked to a history of smoking • Tends to be found centrally, near a bronchus	• Can appear in any part of the lung • Tends to grow and spread quickly

The remaining 20% of lung cancers are small-cell lung cancer. Although the cancer cells in this type of cancer are small, they can multiply quickly and form large tumors that spread to the lymph nodes and other structures, such as the brain, liver, and bones.

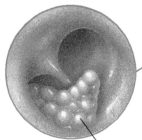

Bronchoscopic view

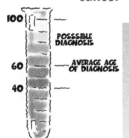

age-old story

Age and lung cancer

100 ⎯ POSSSIBLE DIAGNOSIS

60 ⎯ AVERAGE AGE OF DIAGNOSIS

40 ⎯

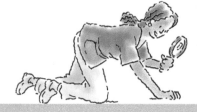

Tumor projecting into bronchi

How it happens

Lung cancer most commonly results from repeated tissue trauma from inhalation of irritants or carcinogens.

Almost all lung cancers start in the epithelium of the lungs. In normal lungs, the epithelium lines and protects the tissue below it. However, when exposed to irritants or carcinogens, the epithelium continually replaces itself until the cells develop chromosomal changes and become dysplastic (altered in size, shape, and organization).

Dysplastic cells don't function well as protectors, so underlying tissue becomes exposed to irritants and carcinogens. Eventually, the dysplastic cells turn into neoplastic carcinoma and start invading deeper tissues.

What to look for

• Cough
• Hoarseness
• Wheezing
• Dyspnea
• Hemoptysis (blood in sputum)
• Chest pain
• Weight loss
• Weakness
• Anorexia
• Dysphagia

Tumor infiltration

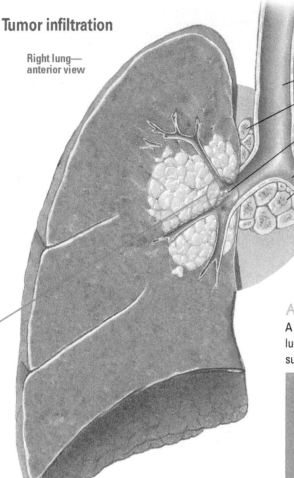

Right lung—
anterior view

Trachea

Metastasis to hilar
lymph nodes

Tumor projecting into
bronchi

Bronchus

Metastasis to carinal
lymph nodes

Adenocarcinoma of the lung

A peripheral tumor in the upper right lobe of the
lung has an irregular border and a tan or gray cut
surface.

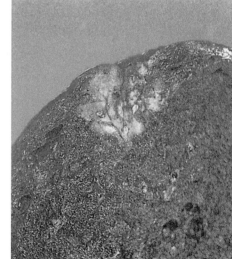

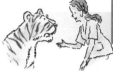

Risk factors for lung cancer

- Exposure to tobacco smoke (including secondhand exposure)
- Exposure to air pollutants, such as asbestos, uranium, arsenic,
nickel, iron oxides, chromium, radioactive dust, coal dust, and radon
- Familial susceptibility

Pneumonia

Pneumonia is an acute infection of the lung parenchyma that commonly impairs gas exchange.

It occurs in both genders and at all ages. More than 4 million cases of pneumonia occur annually in the United States. It's the leading cause of death from infectious disease.

The prognosis is good for patients with normal lungs and adequate immune systems. However, bacterial pneumonia is the leading cause of death in debilitated patients.

How it happens

In bacterial pneumonia, an infection triggers alveolar inflammation and edema. An exudative fluid builds up between the alveoli and capillaries, which obstructs transfer of oxygen to blood.

In viral pneumonia, the virus attacks bronchial epithelial cells, causing inflammation and desquamation. The virus also invades mucous glands and goblet cells, spreading to the alveoli, which fill with blood and fluid.

risky business

Risk factors for pneumonia

- Chronic illness and debilitation
- Cancer (particularly lung cancer)
- Abdominal and thoracic surgery
- Atelectasis
- Colds or other viral respiratory infections
- Chronic respiratory disease, such as COPD, bronchiectasis, or cystic fibrosis
- Influenza
- Smoking
- Malnutrition
- Alcoholism
- Sickle cell disease
- Tracheostomy
- Exposure to noxious gases
- Aspiration
- Immunosuppressive therapy
- Premature birth

Classifications

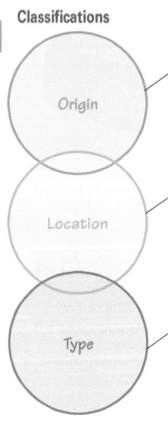

Origin

Pneumonia may be viral, bacterial, fungal, or protozoal in origin.

Location

Bronchopneumonia involves distal airways and alveoli; lobular pneumonia, part of a lobe; and lobar pneumonia, an entire lobe.

Type

Primary pneumonia results from inhalation or aspiration of a pathogen, such as bacteria or a virus, and includes pneumococcal and viral pneumonia; *secondary* pneumonia may follow lung damage from a noxious chemical or other insult or may result from hematogenous spread of bacteria; *aspiration* pneumonia results from aspiration of vomitus or food particles into the bronchi instead of the esophagus.

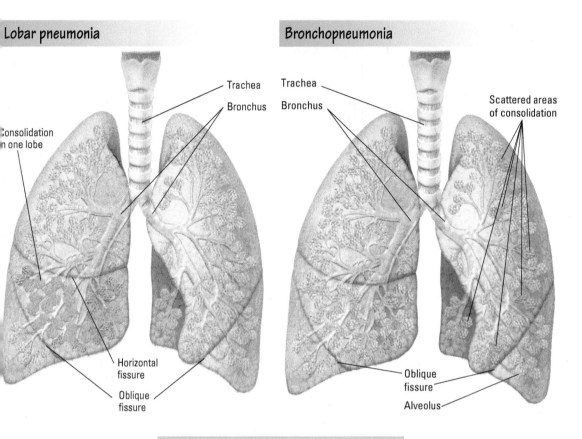

Lobar pneumonia

Trachea

Bronchus

Consolidation in one lobe

Horizontal fissure

Oblique fissure

Bronchopneumonia

Trachea

Bronchus

Scattered areas of consolidation

Oblique fissure

Alveolus

What to look for

- Fever
- Pleuritic pain
- Chills
- Malaise
- Tachypnea
- Dyspnea
- Cough with purulent, yellow, or bloody sputum
- Crackles
- Decreased breath sounds

Pneumothorax

Pneumothorax is an accumulation of air in the pleural cavity that leads to partial or complete lung collapse. The most common types of pneumothorax are open, closed, and tension.

Now that's what I call a collapse!

How it happens

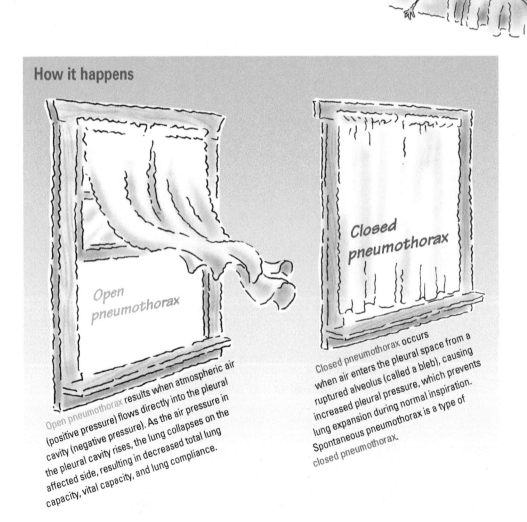

Open pneumothorax

Open pneumothorax results when atmospheric air (positive pressure) flows directly into the pleural cavity (negative pressure). As the air pressure in the pleural cavity rises, the lung collapses on the affected side, resulting in decreased total lung capacity, vital capacity, and lung compliance.

Closed pneumothorax

Closed pneumothorax occurs when air enters the pleural space from a ruptured alveolus (called a bleb), causing increased pleural pressure, which prevents lung expansion during normal inspiration. Spontaneous pneumothorax is a type of closed pneumothorax.

Open pneumothorax

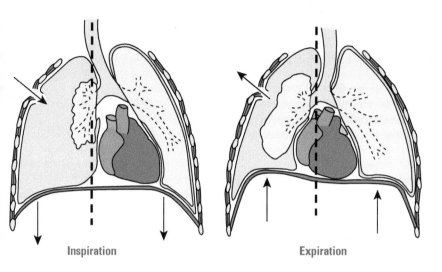

Inspiration   **Expiration**

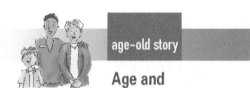

age-old story

Age and pneumothorax

Spontaneous pneumothorax is common in older patients with chronic pulmonary disease, but it may also occur in healthy, tall young adults.

Closed pneumothorax

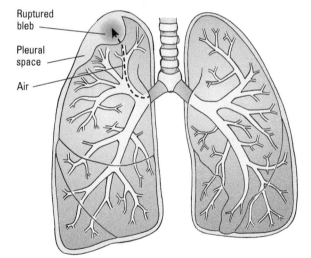

Ruptured bleb

Pleural space

Air

Tension pneumothorax results when air in the pleural space is under higher pressure than air in the adjacent lung. The air enters the pleural space from the site of pleural rupture, which acts as a one-way valve. Air is allowed to enter into the pleural space on inspiration but can't escape as the rupture site closes on expiration. More air enters on inspiration, and air pressure begins to exceed barometric pressure. Increasing air pressure pushes against the recoiled lung, causing compression atelectasis.

As air continues to accumulate and intrapleural pressures increase, the mediastinum shifts away from the affected side and decreases venous return. This forces the heart, trachea, esophagus, and great vessels to the unaffected side, compressing the heart and the contralateral lung.

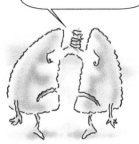

I'm in high distress. Closed pneumothorax can't be far behind!

Tension pneumothorax

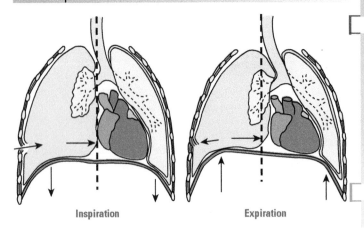

Inspiration   Expiration

What to look for

Closed pneumothorax
- Sudden, sharp, pleuritic pain exacerbated by chest movement, breathing, and coughing
- Asymmetrical chest wall movement
- Shortness of breath
- Cyanosis
- Hyperresonance or tympany heard with percussion
- Respiratory distress

Open pneumothorax
- Signs and symptoms of closed pneumothorax
- Absent breath sounds on the affected side
- Chest rigidity on the affected side
- Tachycardia
- Crackling beneath the skin on palpation

Tension pneumothorax
- Decreased cardiac output
- Hypotension
- Compensatory tachycardia
- Tachypnea
- Lung collapse
- Mediastinal shift and tracheal deviation to the opposite side
- Cardiac arrest

Pulmonary edema

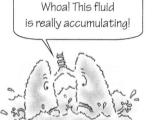

Whoa! This fluid is really accumulating!

Pulmonary edema is a common complication of cardiac disorders. It's marked by accumulated fluid in the interstitial spaces of the lung. It may occur as a chronic condition or develop quickly and rapidly become fatal.

A closer look

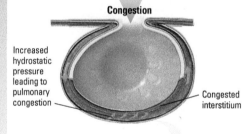

Normal

Capillary

Alveolus

Interstitial space

Hydrostatic pressure pushes fluids into the interstitial space.

Plasma oncotic pressure pulls fluids back into the bloodstream.

Congestion

Increased hydrostatic pressure leading to pulmonary congestion

Congested interstitium

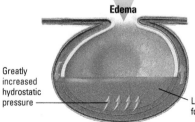

Edema

Greatly increased hydrostatic pressure

Large amount of fluid forced into the alveolus

How it happens

Pulmonary edema commonly results from left-sided heart failure. In left-sided heart failure, blood volume accumulates in the left ventricle because the ventricle is too weak to push it forward into the aorta. High blood volume in the left ventricle causes high hydrostatic pressure backward into the left atrium. Hydrostatic pressure then builds up backward into the pulmonary veins and pulmonary capillaries. The high hydrostatic pressure in the capillaries causes fluid from the blood to push out into the pulmonary interstitial spaces, causing pulmonary edema. The fluid blocks oxygen diffusion into the capillaries causing hypoxia.

What to look for

Early
* Exertional dyspnea
* Paroxysmal nocturnal dyspnea
* Orthopnea
* Cough
* Mild tachypnea
* Pulmonary crackles
* Tachycardia

Late
* Labored, rapid respiration
* Orthopnea; need to sit straight up to breathe
* Diffuse course crackles
* Cough producing frothy, bloody sputum
* Increased tachycardia
* Arrhythmias
* Cold, clammy skin
* Diaphoresis
* Cyanosis
* Decreased blood pressure
* Thready pulse

Pulmonary embolism

Pulmonary embolism is an obstruction of the pulmonary arterial bed by a dislodged thrombus, heart valve growths, or a foreign substance. A thrombus commonly travels up into the right side of the heart from the deep veins in the lower extremity. The thrombus lodges in the pulmonary arterial circulation.

Pulmonary perfusion decreases causing pulmonary ischemia and pulmonary infarction leading to decreased transfer of oxygen from alveoli into capillaries.

Although pulmonary infarction that results from embolism may be so mild as to produce no symptoms, massive embolism (more than a 50% obstruction of pulmonary arterial circulation) and the accompanying infarction can be rapidly fatal.

How it happens

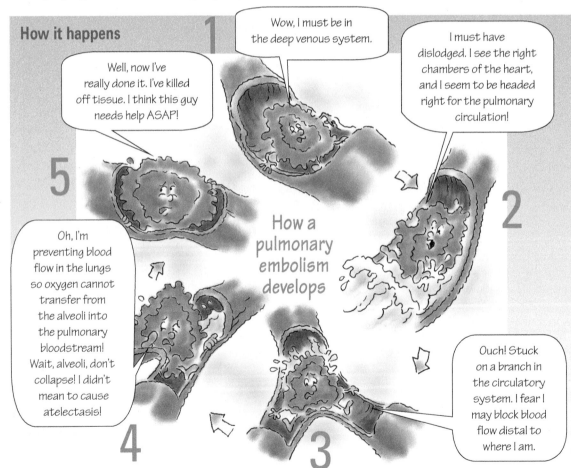

How a pulmonary embolism develops

What to look for

Common
- Dyspnea
- Anginal or pleuritic chest pain
- Tachycardia
- Productive cough (sputum may be blood tinged)
- Pleural effusion

Less common
- Massive hemoptysis
- Splinting of the chest
- Leg edema
- Cyanosis
- Syncope
- Pleural friction rub
- Weak, rapid pulse
- Hypotension
- Restlessness
- Anxiety

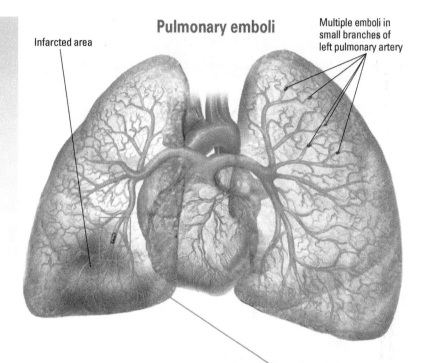

Pulmonary emboli

Infarcted area

Multiple emboli in small branches of left pulmonary artery

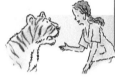

risky business

Risk factors for pulmonary embolism

- Chronic pulmonary disease
- Heart failure or atrial fibrillation
- Recent surgery
- Deep venous thrombosis (DVT)
- Vascular injury
- Venous stasis
- Increased blood coagulability
- Long-term immobility
- Use of hormonal contraceptives
- Obesity
- Pregnancy

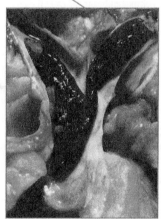

Large, solid embolus

Severe acute respiratory syndrome

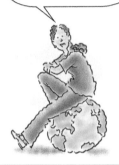

The World Health Organization stated that 8,098 people became ill with SARS during the 2003 outbreak. Of those, 774 died.

Severe acute respiratory syndrome (SARS) is a viral respiratory tract infection that can progress to pneumonia and, eventually, death.

The disease was first recognized in 2003 with outbreaks in China, Canada, Singapore, Taiwan, and Vietnam, with other countries—including the United States—reporting smaller numbers of cases. During the 2003 outbreak, SARS was found to be less common among children and to be milder in form in this age-group when it did occur.

How it happens

The SARS virus incubates for 2 to 10 days. SARS is thought to be transmitted by respiratory droplets produced when an infected person coughs or sneezes. The droplets are propelled a short distance (typically up to 3 feet) through the air and deposited on the mucous membranes of the mouth, nose, or eyes of a person who's nearby. The virus can also spread when a person touches a surface or object contaminated with infectious droplets and then touches the mouth, nose, or eyes.

The SARS virion (A) attaches to receptors on the host cell membrane and releases enzymes (called *absorption*) (B) that weaken the membrane and enable the SARS virion to penetrate the cell. The SARS virion removes the protein coating that protects its genetic material (C), replicates (D), and matures and then escapes from the host cell by budding from the plasma membrane (E). The infection then can spread to other host cells.

What to look for

Stage 1
* Fever (greater than 100.4°F [38°C])
* Fatigue
* Headache
* Chills
* Myalgia
* Malaise
* Anorexia
* Diarrhea

Stage 2
* Dry cough
* Dyspnea
* Progressive hypoxemia
* Respiratory failure

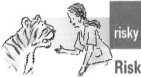

risky business

Risk factors for SAR

* Close contact with an infected person
* Contact with aerosolized (exhaled) droplets and bod secretions from an infected person
* Travel to endemic areas

Tuberculosis

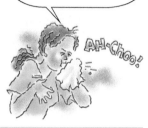

Use tissues to limit those droplets that are responsible for transmitting TB.

Tuberculosis (TB) is an acute or chronic mycobacterium infection characterized by pulmonary infiltrates and the formation of granulomas with caseation, fibrosis, and cavitation. The main site of infection is the lung, but approximately 15% of infections are extrapulmonary.

How it happens

Multiplication of the bacillus *Mycobacterium tuberculosis* causes an inflammatory process.

A cell-mediated (T-cell) immune response follows that usually contains the infection within 4 to 6 weeks. The T-cell response results in the formation of granulomas around the bacilli, making them dormant. Bacilli within granulomas may remain viable for many years, resulting in a positive purified protein derivative (PPD) or other skin tests for TB. A blood test can also be done to diagnose TB.

Active disease develops in 5% to 15% of those infected with *M. tuberculosis*. Transmission occurs when an infected person coughs or sneezes, which spreads infected droplets.

Primary TB

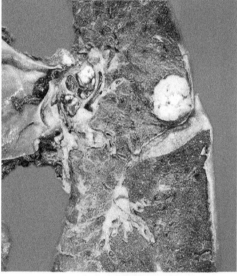

What to look for

* Fatigue
* Cough
* Fever
* Night sweats
* Anorexia
* Weight loss
* Chest pain
* Blood-tinged sputum
* Dullness over the affected area
* Crepitant crackles
* Bronchial breath sounds
* Wheezes
* Whispered pectoriloquy (sound heard through the stethoscope when the patient whispers a word or number)

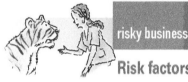

risky business

Risk factors for TB

* Close contact with a newly diagnosed patient
* History of previous TB exposure
* Recent emigration or travel (from Africa, Asia, Mexico, or South America)
* History of silicosis, diabetes, malnutrition, cancer, Hodgkin disease, or leukemia
* Drug or alcohol abuse
* Residence in a nursing home, mental health facility, or prison
* Immunosuppression or corticosteroid use
* Homelessness
* HIV

Upper respiratory tract infection

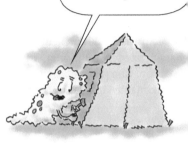

Well, this looks like as good a place as any to set up camp for a few weeks and see if I can stir up a secondary infection.

Upper respiratory tract infection (also known as the *common cold* or *acute coryza*) is an acute, usually afebrile viral infection that causes inflammation of the upper respiratory tract. It's the most common infectious disease. Although a cold is benign and self-limiting, it can lead to secondary bacterial infections.

How it happens

Infection occurs when the offending organism gains entry into the upper respiratory tract, proliferates, and begins an inflammatory reaction. As a result, acute inflammation of the upper airway structures, including the sinuses, nasopharynx, pharynx, larynx, and trachea, occurs.

The presence of the pathogen triggers infiltration of the mucous membranes by inflammatory and infection-fighting cells. Mucosal swelling and secretion of a serous or mucopurulent exudate result.

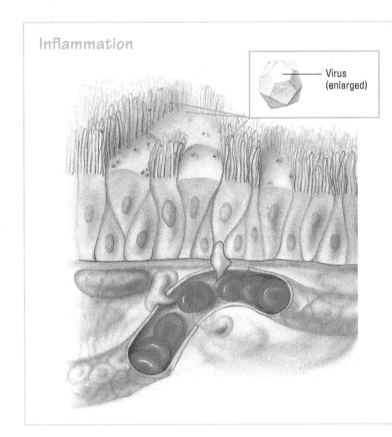

Inflammation

Virus (enlarged)

What to look for

- Pharyngitis
- Nasal congestion
- Coryza (acute rhinitis)
- Sneezing
- Headache
- Burning, watery eyes
- Fever
- Chills
- Myalgia
- Arthralgia
- Malaise
- Lethargy
- Hacking, nonproductive, or nocturnal cough

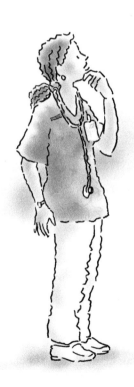

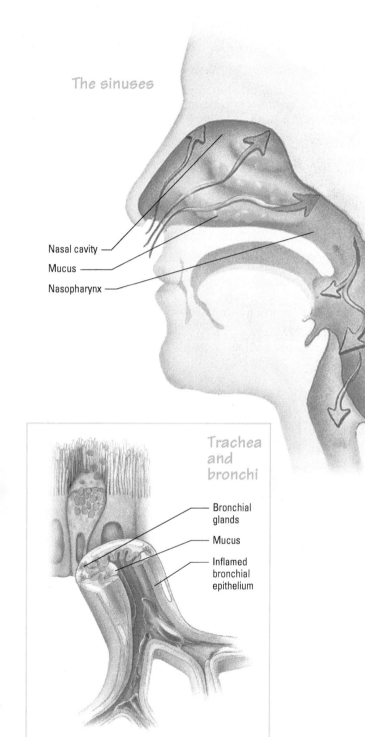

The sinuses

Nasal cavity

Mucus

Nasopharynx

Trachea and bronchi

Bronchial glands

Mucus

Inflamed bronchial epithelium

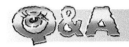

My word!

Solve the word scrambles to uncover terms related to respiratory disorders. Then, rearrange the circled letters from those words to answer the question posed.

1. horapntomxeu _____◯◯_____

2. crisinbhot _____◯

3. nelaznuif _____◯

4. ymseaphme _◯_____◯

Answer: _____

Show and tell

Identify the types of pneumothorax in these illustrations and describe each.

Question: What condition discussed in this chapter is considered to be a chronic obstructive pulmonary disease?

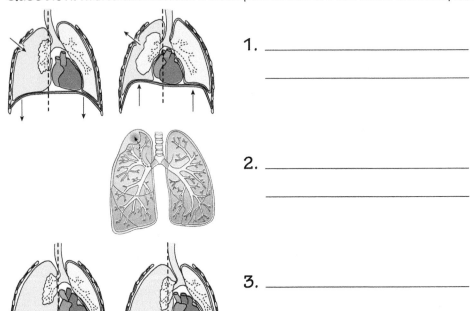

1. _____

_____

2. _____

_____

3. _____

_____

Selected References

Centers for Disease Control and Prevention. (2014, September 9). Key facts about influenza. Retrieved from: http://www.cdc.gov/flu/keyfacts.htm

Centers for Disease Control and Prevention. (2015, April 23). National current asthma prevalence. Retrieved from: http://www.cdc.gov/asthma/most_recent_data.htm

Centers for Disease Control and Prevention. (2015, July 22). Severe acute respiratory syndrome. Retrieved from: http://www.cdc.gov/sars/index.html

Earwood, J. S., & Thompson, T. D. (2015). Hemoptysis: Evaluation and management. *American Family Physician, 91*(4), 243–249.

Erlikh, I. V., Abraham, S., & Kondamudi, V. K. (2010). Management of influenza. *American Family Physician, 82*(9), 1087–1095.

Fashner, J., Ericson, K., & Werner, S. (2012). Treatment of the common cold in children and adults. *American Family Physician, 86*(2), 153–159.

Hopkins, T. G., Maher, E. R., Reid, E., & Marciniak, S. J. (2011). Recurrent pneumothorax. *Lancet, 377*(9777), 1624.

Kumar, V., Abbas, A., & Aster, J. (2015). *Robbins & Cotran pathologic basis of disease* (9th ed.). Philadelphia, PA: Elsevier-Saunders.

Latimer, K. M., & Mott, T. F. (2015). Lung cancer: Diagnosis, treatment principles, and screening. *American Family Physician, 91*(4), 250–256.

Medline Plus, US National Library of Medicine. (2014, February 2). Acute respiratory distress syndrome. Retrieved from: http://www.nlm.nih.gov/medlineplus/ency/article/000103.htm

National Heart Lung and Blood Institute. (2011, July 1). Who is at risk for pulmonary embolism? Retrieved from http://www.nhlbi.nih.gov/health/health-topics/topics/pe/atrisk

Okpapi, A., Friend, A. J., & Turner, S. W. (2013). Acute asthma and other recurrent wheezing disorders in children. *American Family Physician, 88*(2), 130–131.

Wahls, S. A. (2012). Causes and evaluation of chronic dyspnea. *American Family Physician, 86*(2), 173–182.

Watkins, R. R., & Lemonovich, T. L. (2011). Diagnosis and management of community-acquired pneumonia in adults. *American Family Physician, 83*(11), 1299–1306.

Chapter 4

Neurologic disorders

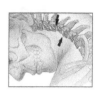

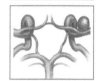
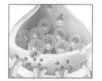

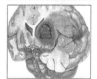
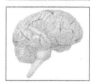
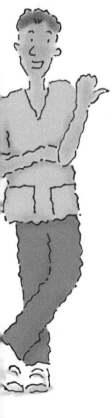

Acceleration–deceleration cervical injury

Neurologic

Acceleration-deceleration cervical injuries (commonly known as *whiplash*) result from sharp hyperextension and flexion of the neck that damage muscles, ligaments, disks, and nerve tissue. The prognosis for this type of injury is usually excellent; symptoms usually subside when treated.

How it happens

...and all of a sudden, BAM—the guy didn't even slow down. I know it's a cervical injury. I can just feel it!

Whiplash injuries of the head and neck

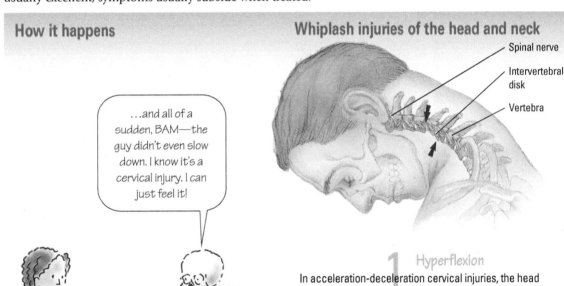

- Spinal nerve
- Intervertebral disk
- Vertebra

1 Hyperflexion

In acceleration-deceleration cervical injuries, the head is propelled in a forward and downward motion in hyperflexion. A wedge-shaped deformity of the bone may be created if the anterior portions of the vertebra are crushed.

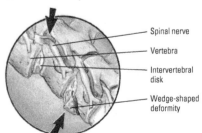

- Spinal nerve
- Vertebra
- Intervertebral disk
- Wedge-shaped deformity

What to look for

- Moderate-to-severe anterior and posterior neck pain
- Dizziness and gait disturbances
- Vomiting
- Headache
- Nuchal rigidity
- Neck muscle asymmetry
- Rigidity or numbness in the arms

Signs and symptoms may develop immediately or may be completely delayed 12 to 24 hours in mild injury.

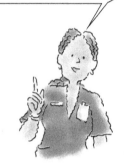

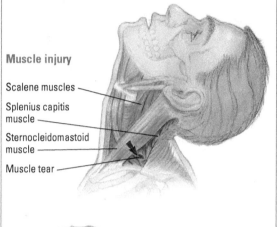

Muscle injury

Scalene muscles

Splenius capitis muscle

Sternocleidomastoid muscle

Muscle tear

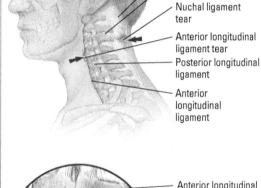

Ligament injury

Nuchal ligament

Interspinous ligament

Nuchal ligament tear

Anterior longitudinal ligament tear

Posterior longitudinal ligament

Anterior longitudinal ligament

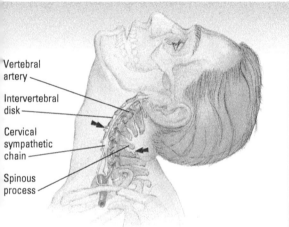

Vertebral artery

Intervertebral disk

Cervical sympathetic chain

Spinous process

 Hyperextension

Then, the head is forced backward in hyperextension. A tear in the anterior ligament may pull pieces of bone from the cervical vertebrae. Spinous processes of the vertebrae may be fractured. Intervertebral disks may be compressed posteriorly and torn anteriorly. Vertebral arteries may be stretched, pinched, or torn, causing reduced blood flow to the brain. Nerves of the cervical sympathetic chain may also be injured.

Injuries of the neck muscles may range from minor strains and microhemorrhages to severe tears.

Anterior longitudinal ligament

Intervertebral disk

Vertebra

Interspinous ligament

Posterior longitudinal ligament

Alzheimer disease

Alzheimer disease is a progressive, degenerative disorder of the cerebral cortex. Cortical degeneration is most marked in the frontal lobes, but atrophy occurs in all areas of the cortex.

Because Alzheimer disease accounts for more than one-half of all dementia cases, I'm trying to keep my mind active!

How it happens

The cause of Alzheimer disease is unknown, but there are contributing factors:
1. Neurochemical factors: deficiency in the neurotransmitter acetylcholine or abnormal amount of glutamate.
2. Genetic factors: gene encoding the cholesterol-carrying apolipoprotein E (*APOE*) on chromosome 19 has been linked to increased risk for AD.

age-old story

Age and Alzheimer disease

Although Alzheimer disease primarily occurs in the elderly population, 1% to 10% of Alzheimer cases have their onset in middle age.

Neurofilament

Dendrites

Nucleus

Cell body

Vacuole

Axon

Message

Tissue changes in Alzheimer disease

Granulovacuolar degeneration

Vacuoles

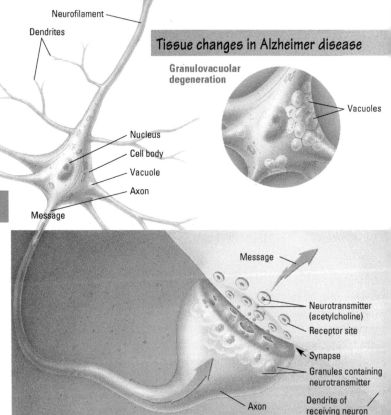

Message

Neurotransmitter (acetylcholine)

Receptor site

Synapse

Granules containing neurotransmitter

Dendrite of receiving neuron

Axon

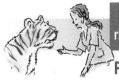

risky business

Risk factors for Alzheimer disease

Risk factors for developing Alzheimer disease are age and a family history of the disease. Having a parent or a sibling with the disease makes you two to three times more at risk for developing the disease than if you didn't have a parent or sibling with the disease.

Other risk factors:

- Advancing age
- APOE 4 genotype
- Obesity
- Insulin resistance
- Vascular factors
- Dyslipidemia
- Hypertension
- Inflammatory markers
- Down syndrome
- Traumatic brain injury
- Depression
- Aluminum toxicity

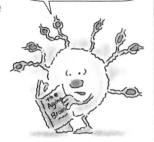

The age of neurons like me seems to play a role in Alzheimer's.

What to look for

Early
- Forgetfulness
- Subtle memory loss without loss of social skills or behavior patterns
- Difficulty learning and retaining new information
- Inability to concentrate
- Deterioration in personal hygiene and appearance

Progressive
- Difficulty with abstract thinking and activities that require judgment
- Progressive difficulty in communicating
- Severe deterioration of memory, language, and motor function progressing to coordination loss and the inability to speak or write
- Repetitive actions
- Restlessness
- Irritability, depression, mood swings, paranoia, hostility, and combativeness
- Nocturnal awakenings
- Disorientation

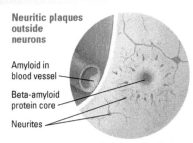

Neurofibrillar tangles in the neuron

Tangles

Neuritic plaques outside neurons

Amyloid in blood vessel

Beta-amyloid protein core

Neurites

Neurofibrillary tangles are twisted fibers mainly consisting of **tau protein** that build up inside neurons and render them dysfunctional.
Neuritic plaques outside neurons: Plaques are dense deposits of the **protein beta-amyloid**.
Cerebrospinal fluid: excessive amounts of **tau protein** found.

This is the one time you don't want to get an A.

I can't remember whether I'm unable to concentrate because of a disorder or because this feels so good!

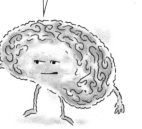

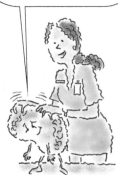

memory board

5 As of DEMENTIA:

Amnesia: memory loss, particularly short-term memory
Agnosia: forgetting purpose of familiar objects in environment
Apraxia: forgetting how to perform familiar activities
Apathy: lack of concern for lost abilities
Aphasia: lack of sensible speech or being mute

Cerebral aneurysm

In an intracranial or cerebral aneurysm, a weakness in the wall of the cerebral artery causes localized dilation. Cerebral aneurysms usually arise at an arterial junction in the circle of Willis, the circular anastomosis connecting the major cerebral arteries at the base of the brain. Many cerebral aneurysms rupture, causing a subarachnoid hemorrhage.

> Cerebral aneurysms are generally asymptomatic until they rupture. Look out!

How it happens

Prolonged hemodynamic stress and local arterial degeneration at vessel bifurcations are believed to be major contributing factors in the development and eventual rupture of cerebral aneurysms.

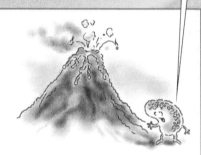

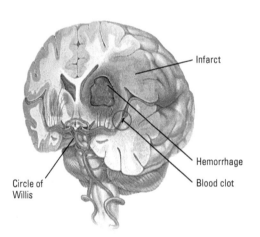

Infarct

Hemorrhage

Blood clot

Circle of Willis

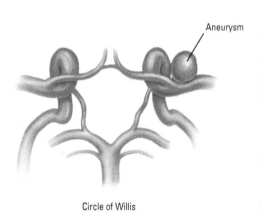

Aneurysm

Circle of Willis

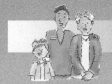

Age and cerebral aneurysm

Incidence is slightly higher in women than in men, especially those in their late 40s or early to mid-50s. However, a cerebral aneurysm may occur at any age and in either gender.

Berry aneurysm

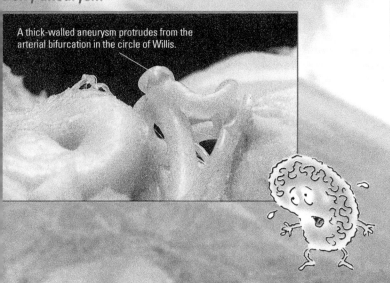

A thick-walled aneurysm protrudes from the arterial bifurcation in the circle of Willis.

What to look for

Subarachnoid hemorrhage
- Change in the level of consciousness
- Sudden severe headache
- Cranial nerve deficits

Depression

Clinical depression is a serious medical condition that affects thoughts, mood, feelings, behavior, and physical health. It's a persistent condition and can interfere significantly with an individual's ability to function. Clinical depression includes dysthymia, major depression, premenstrual dysmorphic disorder, postpartum depression, and seasonal affective disorder.

The role of neurotransmitters

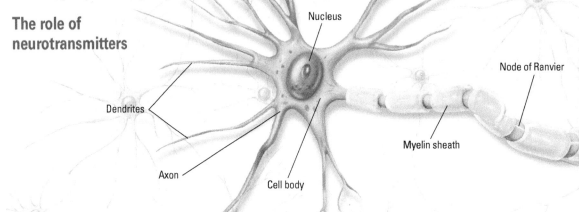

Nucleus

Node of Ranvier

Dendrites

Myelin sheath

Axon

Cell body

How it happens

Neurotransmitters are chemical messengers released into the synapses (gaps) between neurons that carry messages from one neuron (nerve cell) to another and affect behavior, mood, and thought. Norepinephrine and serotonin are two of the neurotransmitters that play a role in depression. Low levels of these neurotransmitters in areas of the brain that control mood and emotion may result in depression.

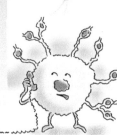

I'd like to send a chemical message, please.

age-old story

Age and depression

The peak age for the onset of depression is between ages 20 and 40. In children, signs and symptoms of depression include hyperactivity, poor school performance, somatic complaints, sleeping and eating disturbances, lack of playfulness, and suicidal ideation or actions.

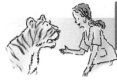

Risk factors for depression

- Stress
- Emotional trauma
- Death of a family member
- Family history of mood disorders, depression, or bipolar disorder
- Cancer, stroke, diabetes, heart disease
- Low self-esteem
- Tobacco use
- Alcohol misuse
- Excess weight

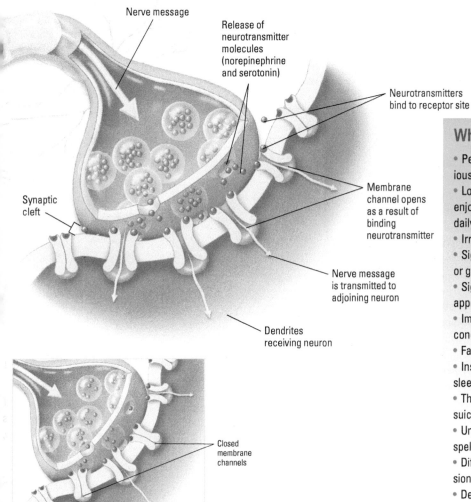

Nerve message

Release of neurotransmitter molecules (norepinephrine and serotonin)

Neurotransmitters bind to receptor site

Synaptic cleft

Membrane channel opens as a result of binding neurotransmitter

Nerve message is transmitted to adjoining neuron

Dendrites receiving neuron

Closed membrane channels

What to look for

- Persistent sad, anxious, or hopeless mood
- Loss of interest or enjoyment in normal daily activities
- Irritability or agitation
- Significant weight loss or gain
- Significant changes in appetite
- Impaired thinking or concentration
- Fatigue
- Insomnia or excessive sleeping
- Thoughts of death or suicide
- Unexplained crying spells
- Difficulty making decisions
- Decreased sex drive

Migraine headache

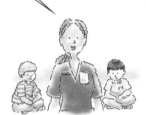

Migraines can first appear in childhood. Pay attention to the symptoms so you can classify the type.

A migraine headache is a throbbing, vascular headache that usually first appears in childhood and commonly recurs throughout adulthood. It may be classified according to the presence of an aura (temporary focal neurologic signs, usually visual), such as scotoma (an area of lost vision in the visual field),

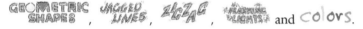 GEOMETRIC SHAPES, JAGGED LINES, ZIGZAG, FLASHING LIGHTS and colors.

A common migraine may not have an aura, whereas a classic migraine has an aura. Migraine headache is more common in women and has a strong familial incidence.

How it happens

The cause of migraine is unclear, however it is believed that prostaglandins, platelets, vascular changes and fluctuations in serotonin level are involved. Prostaglandin, a hormone present in the bloodstream, signals the platelets to aggregate. Platelet aggregation causes the release of serotonin (a chemical that transmits signals to nerves).

This increase in serotonin causes nerves to signal the blood vessels to vasoconstrict or decrease in diameter, which, in turn, causes a decrease in blood flow (ischemia) around the brain. This localized ischemia causes an increase in acid (acidosis). The localized acidosis and ischemia cause blood vessels to dilate.

Vasodilation of the innervated arteries results in the headache phase. Inflammation to the surrounding vessels may prolong the headache pain.

Platelet aggregation then decreases, lowering the serotonin level, which results in vasodilation. A painful inflammation occurs around the surrounding areas, which can persist.

Theory for the migraine

Normal blood vessel with hormone in bloodstream

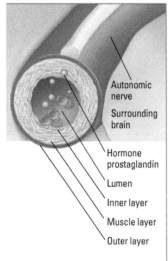

Autonomic nerve

Surrounding brain

Hormone prostaglandin

Lumen

Inner layer

Muscle layer

Outer layer

Constricted blood vessel

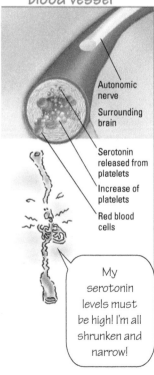

Autonomic nerve

Surrounding brain

Serotonin released from platelets

Increase of platelets

Red blood cells

My serotonin levels must be high! I'm all shrunken and narrow!

Age and migraines

In children, a common symptom of a migraine headache is intense nausea and vomiting, which may be associated with abdominal pain and fever.

The pathways of a migraine

Electrical impulses spread to other regions of the brain.

Chemicals in the brain cause blood vessel dilation and inflammation of surrounding tissue.

Changes in nerve cell activity and blood flow may result in such symptoms as vision disturbances, numbness or tingling, and dizziness.

4

3

2

1

5

Migraine originates deep within the brain.

Dilated blood vessel

Perivascular inflammation from surrounding brain

Decrease of platelets

Red blood cells

Trigeminal nerve ganglion and nuclei

The inflammation irritates the trigeminal nerve, resulting in severe or throbbing pain.

Well, my levels are low. Look how swollen I am! I'm at risk for a migraine!

What to look for

- Auras
- Unilateral in onset but may become generalized
- Begins as a dull ache that progresses into throbbing, pulsating one-sided pain
- Photophobia (sensitivity to light)
- Nausea and vomiting
- Paresthesia
- Phonophobia (sensitivity to sound)

Multiple sclerosis

Multiple sclerosis (MS) results from progressive demyelination of the white matter of the brain and spinal cord, leading to widespread neurologic dysfunction. The structures usually involved are the optic and oculomotor nerves, cerebellum, and the spinal nerve tracts. It is characterized by exacerbations and remissions.

How it happens

The exact cause of MS is unknown. It is theorized to be an autoimmune response of the nervous system. Other possible causes include trauma, anoxia, toxins, nutritional deficiencies, vascular lesions, and anorexia nervosa, all of which may help destroy axons and the myelin sheath.

In addition, emotional stress, overwork, fatigue, pregnancy, or an acute respiratory tract infection may precede the onset of MS. Genetic factors may also play a part.

MS affects the white matter of the brain and spinal cord by creating scattered demyelinated lesions that prevent normal neurologic conduction. After the myelin is destroyed, neuroglial tissue in the white matter of the CNS proliferates, forming hard yellow plaques of scar tissue.

Scar tissue damages the underlying axon fiber, disrupting nerve conduction.

Plaque formation

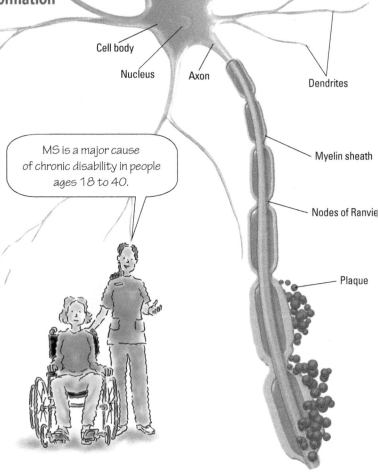

Cell body

Nucleus

Axon

Dendrites

Myelin sheath

Nodes of Ranvier

Plaque

MS is a major cause of chronic disability in people ages 18 to 40.

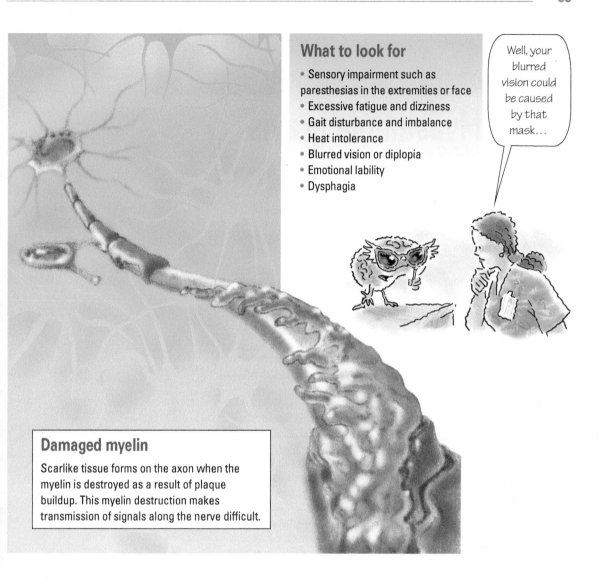

What to look for

- Sensory impairment such as paresthesias in the extremities or face
- Excessive fatigue and dizziness
- Gait disturbance and imbalance
- Heat intolerance
- Blurred vision or diplopia
- Emotional lability
- Dysphagia

Well, your blurred vision could be caused by that mask...

Damaged myelin

Scarlike tissue forms on the axon when the myelin is destroyed as a result of plaque buildup. This myelin destruction makes transmission of signals along the nerve difficult.

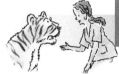

risky business

Risk factors for MS

- Female gender
- Residence in northern urban areas and in higher socioeconomic groups
- Family history of the disease

Myasthenia gravis

Myasthenia gravis produces sporadic, progressive weakness and abnormal fatigue of voluntary skeletal muscles. These effects are exacerbated by exercise and repeated movement.

Myasthenia gravis usually affects muscles in the face, lips, tongue, neck, and throat, which are innervated by the cranial nerves. However, it can affect any muscle group. Eventually, muscle fibers may degenerate, and weakness (especially of the head, neck, trunk, and limb muscles) may become irreversible. When the disease involves the respiratory system, it may be life threatening.

How it happens

Normal neuromuscular transmission

Motor nerve impulses travel to motor nerve terminal.

↓

Acetylcholine (Ach) is released.

↓

Ach diffuses across synapse.

↓

Ach receptor sites in motor end plates depolarize muscle fiber.

↓

Depolarization spreads, causing muscle contraction.

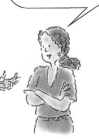

I'm tellin' ya, I'm through with exercise. I don't want myasthenia gravis.

I don't think you understand— exercise doesn't cause myasthenia gravis...you just don't want to work out.

Axon

Ach

Ach release site

Normal Ach receptors

Nerve impulses

Motor end plate of muscle

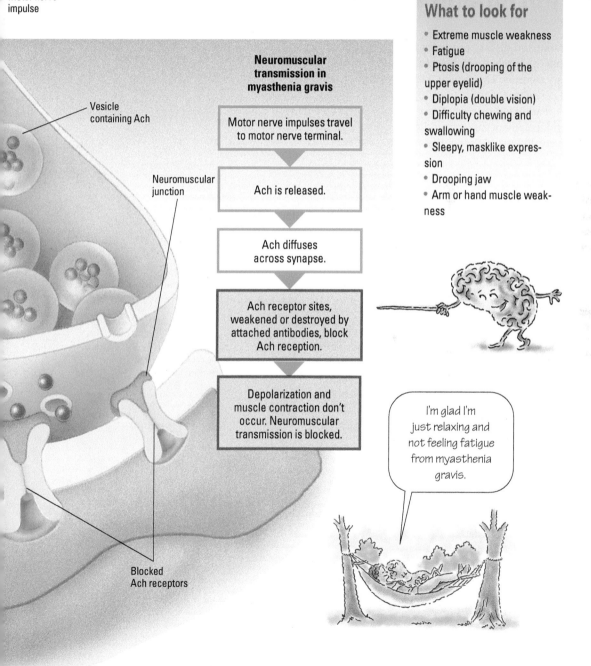

Motor nerve impulse

Vesicle containing Ach

Neuromuscular junction

Blocked Ach receptors

Neuromuscular transmission in myasthenia gravis

Motor nerve impulses travel to motor nerve terminal.

Ach is released.

Ach diffuses across synapse.

Ach receptor sites, weakened or destroyed by attached antibodies, block Ach reception.

Depolarization and muscle contraction don't occur. Neuromuscular transmission is blocked.

What to look for

- Extreme muscle weakness
- Fatigue
- Ptosis (drooping of the upper eyelid)
- Diplopia (double vision)
- Difficulty chewing and swallowing
- Sleepy, masklike expression
- Drooping jaw
- Arm or hand muscle weakness

I'm glad I'm just relaxing and not feeling fatigue from myasthenia gravis.

Parkinson disease

Parkinson disease produces progressive muscle rigidity, loss of muscle movement (akinesia), and involuntary tremors. The patient with Parkinson disease may deteriorate for more than 10 years.

Parkinson disease affects more men than women and usually occurs in middle age or later, striking 1 in every 100 people older than age 60.

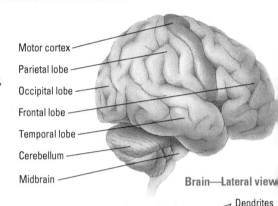

Motor cortex
Parietal lobe
Occipital lobe
Frontal lobe
Temporal lobe
Cerebellum
Midbrain

Brain—Lateral view

How it happens

Parkinson disease affects the extrapyramidal system, which influences the initiation, modulation, and completion of movement. The extrapyramidal system includes the corpus striatum, globus pallidus, and substantia nigra in the midbrain.

In Parkinson disease, a dopamine deficiency occurs in the basal ganglia, the dopamine-releasing pathway that connects the substantia nigra to the corpus striatum.

The normal balance upset prevents affected brain cells from performing their normal inhibitory function within the CNS and causes most parkinsonian symptoms.

Neurotransmitter action in Parkinson disease

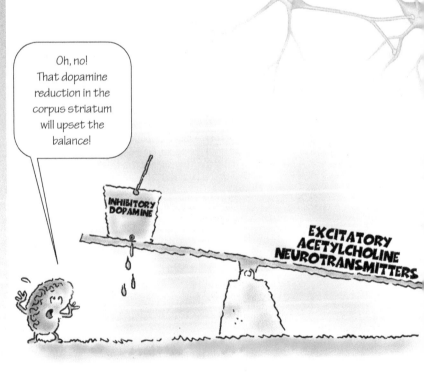

Dendrites

Oh, no! That dopamine reduction in the corpus striatum will upset the balance!

INHIBITORY DOPAMINE

EXCITATORY ACETYLCHOLINE NEUROTRANSMITTERS

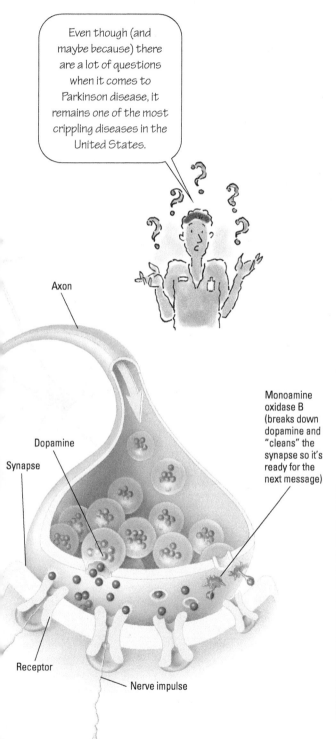

Even though (and maybe because) there are a lot of questions when it comes to Parkinson disease, it remains one of the most crippling diseases in the United States.

Axon

Dopamine

Synapse

Monoamine oxidase B (breaks down dopamine and "cleans" the synapse so it's ready for the next message)

Receptor

Nerve impulse

What to look for

- Bradykinesia (slowed-up movements)
- Muscle rigidity, either uniform (lead-pipe rigidity) or jerky (cogwheel rigidity)
- Akinesia (freezing in place, unable to move)
- A unilateral "pill-rolling," resting tremor
- Gait and movement disturbances
- Masklike facial expression
- Head bobbing

Dopamine levels

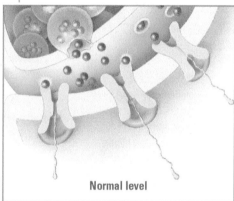

Normal level

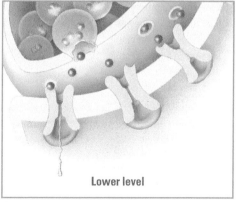

Lower level

Seizure disorder

Seizure disorder (also known as *epilepsy*) is a brain condition characterized by recurrent paroxysmal events associated with abnormal electrical discharges of neurons in the brain. The discharge may trigger a convulsive movement, an interruption of sensation, an alteration in the patient's level of consciousness, or a combination of these symptoms. In most cases, epilepsy doesn't affect intelligence.

It affects people of all ages, races, and ethnic backgrounds; about 2.5 to 3 million people have been diagnosed with epilepsy

How it happens

- The electrical balance at the neuronal level is altered, causing the membrane of the neuron to become easily activated.
- Increased permeability of the membranes helps hypersensitive neurons fire abnormally. Abnormal firing may be activated by hyperthermia, hypoglycemia, hyponatremia, hypoxia, or repeated sensory stimulation.
- When the intensity of a seizure discharge has progressed sufficiently, it spreads to adjacent brain areas. The midbrain, thalamus, and cerebral cortex are most likely to become epileptogenic (producing epileptic attacks).
- Excitement feeds back from the primary focus and to other parts of the brain.
- The discharges become less frequent until they stop.

Seizures

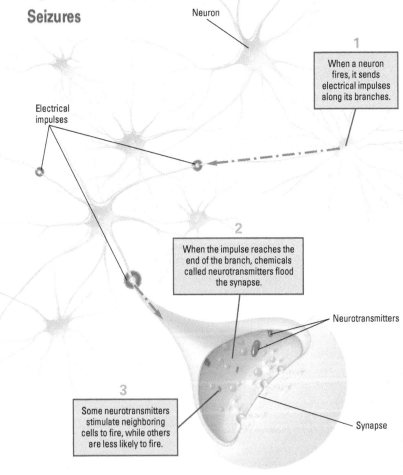

Neuron

1 When a neuron fires, it sends electrical impulses along its branches.

Electrical impulses

2 When the impulse reaches the end of the branch, chemicals called neurotransmitters flood the synapse.

Neurotransmitters

3 Some neurotransmitters stimulate neighboring cells to fire, while others are less likely to fire.

Synapse

Generalized seizures

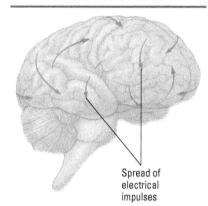

Spread of
electrical
impulses

Generalized seizures occur as the misfiring signals move across both hemispheres. The patient loses consciousness and has body-wide uncontrollable muscle spasms.

Partial seizures

Complex   Simple

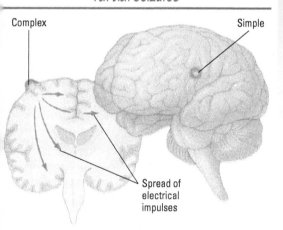

Spread of
electrical
impulses

A *complex-partial seizure* may begin in one hemisphere, but it quickly moves into both hemispheres. The patient commonly stares into space, unaware of the environment. The patient may make purposeless movements.

A *simple-partial seizure* begins in one hemisphere of the brain. One part of the body is usually involved in involuntary movements. The patient doesn't usually lose consciousness.

age-old story

Age and seizures

The incidence of seizure disorder is highest in childhood and old age. The prognosis is good if the patient adheres strictly to the prescribed treatment.

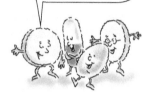

Stick with us, and you'll be in good shape!

What to look for

Auras
- Pungent smell
- Nausea or indigestion
- Rising or sinking feeling in the stomach
- Dreamy feeling
- Unusual taste
- Vision disturbance such as a flashing light

Seizures
- Tonic stiffening followed by muscular contractions
- Tongue biting
- Incontinence
- Blank stare
- Purposeless motor activities
- Changes in level of awareness
- Loss of postural tone
- Jerking and twitching

Oh, good—for a minute there I was worried about a seizure. The pungent smell, the sinking feeling in my stomach, and my indigestion were caused by tonight's dinner. The flashing lights were my premonition of the grease fire.

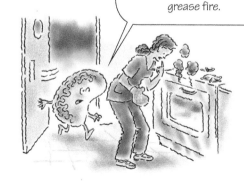

Stroke

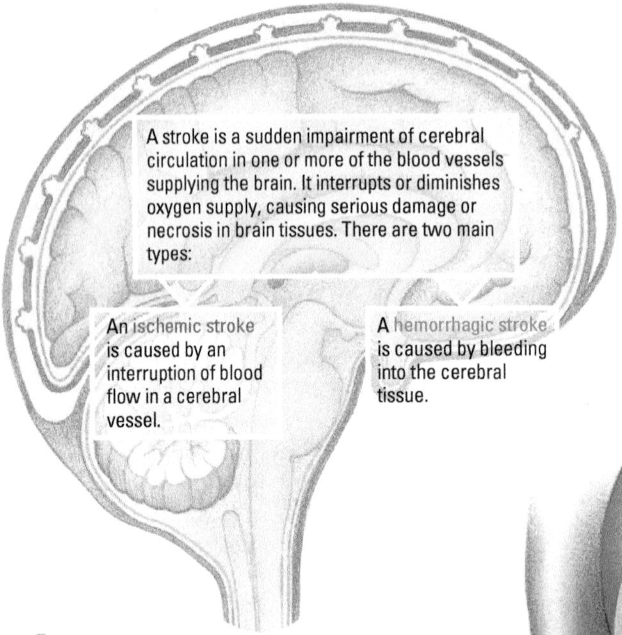

Age and stroke

Although strokes may occur in younger persons, most patients experiencing strokes are older than age 65. In fact, the risk of stroke doubles with each passing decade after age 55.

How it happens

A stroke is a sudden impairment of cerebral circulation in one or more of the blood vessels supplying the brain. It interrupts or diminishes oxygen supply, causing serious damage or necrosis in brain tissues. There are two main types:

An ischemic stroke is caused by an interruption of blood flow in a cerebral vessel.

A hemorrhagic stroke is caused by bleeding into the cerebral tissue.

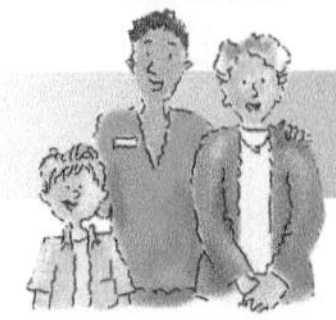

1 Cardiac thromboses develop as a result of various conditions. Emboli break away from their site of origin and move from the heart into the general circulation.

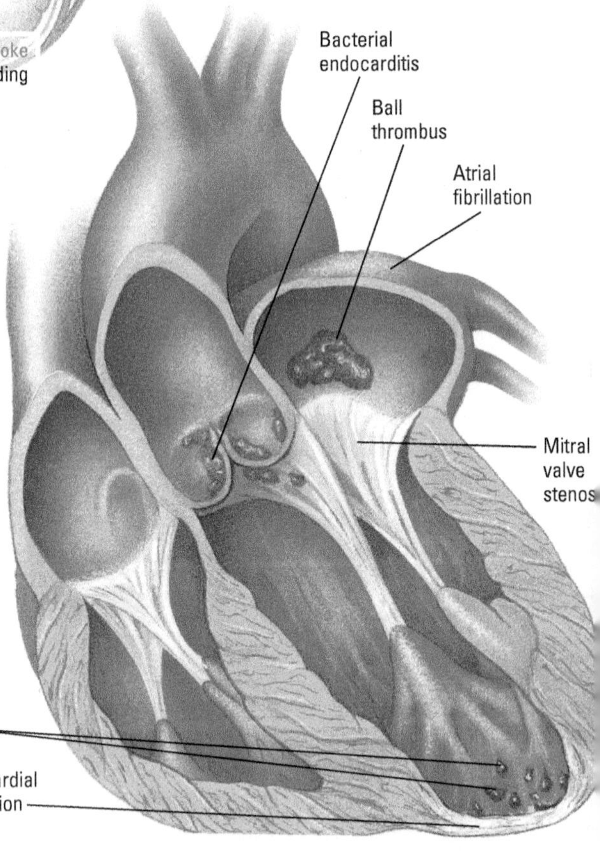

Bacterial endocarditis

Ball thrombus

Atrial fibrillation

Mitral valve stenosis

Mural thrombi

Myocardial infarction

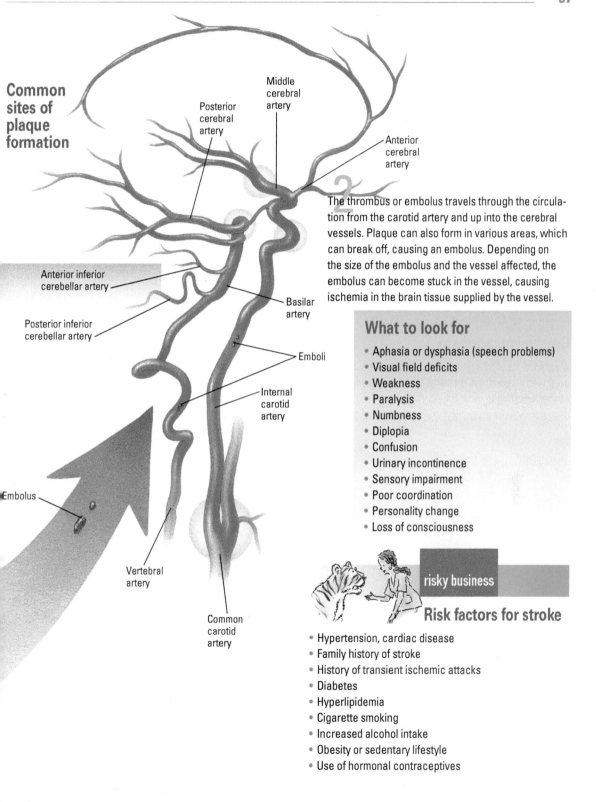

Common sites of plaque formation

Middle cerebral artery

Posterior cerebral artery

Anterior cerebral artery

Anterior inferior cerebellar artery

Posterior inferior cerebellar artery

Basilar artery

Emboli

Internal carotid artery

Embolus

Vertebral artery

Common carotid artery

The thrombus or embolus travels through the circulation from the carotid artery and up into the cerebral vessels. Plaque can also form in various areas, which can break off, causing an embolus. Depending on the size of the embolus and the vessel affected, the embolus can become stuck in the vessel, causing ischemia in the brain tissue supplied by the vessel.

What to look for

- Aphasia or dysphasia (speech problems)
- Visual field deficits
- Weakness
- Paralysis
- Numbness
- Diplopia
- Confusion
- Urinary incontinence
- Sensory impairment
- Poor coordination
- Personality change
- Loss of consciousness

risky business

Risk factors for stroke

- Hypertension, cardiac disease
- Family history of stroke
- History of transient ischemic attacks
- Diabetes
- Hyperlipidemia
- Cigarette smoking
- Increased alcohol intake
- Obesity or sedentary lifestyle
- Use of hormonal contraceptives

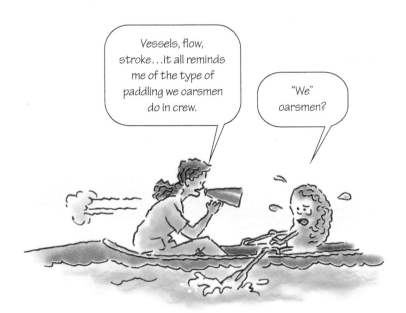

Cerebral hemorrhage

A cerebral hemorrhage can occur like this one, which produced a hematoma that extended into the ventricle, almost rupturing it.

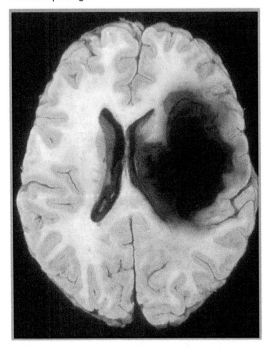

Subarachnoid hemorrhage

Hypertension may cause microaneurysms and tiny arterioles to rupture in the brain, creating pressure on adjacent arterioles and causing them to burst, which leads to more bleeding. Trauma can cause a subarachnoid hemorrhage, which places more pressure on brain tissue.

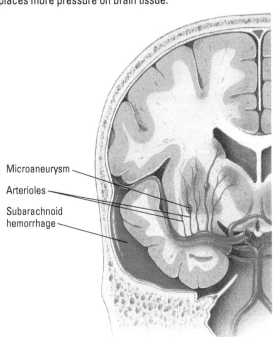

Microaneurysm

Arterioles

Subarachnoid hemorrhage

Meningitis

Meningitis is inflammation of the covering of the brain and spinal cord caused by infection. It usually affects children, but can affect all ages.

How it happens

The inflammation is in response to a viral, bacterial, or other infection of the meninges. Bacterial meningitis is most common and usually follows a respiratory, sinus, or middle ear infection. Common bacteria known to cause meningitis include *Haemophilus influenzae*, *Streptococcus pneumoniae*, and *Neisseria meningitidis*.

　　Children exposed at daycare centers are at a greater risk. Adolescents and young adults who live in dormitories are also at increased risk.

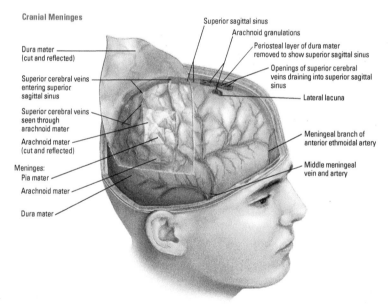

Cranial Meninges

- Dura mater (cut and reflected)
- Superior cerebral veins entering superior sagittal sinus
- Superior cerebral veins seen through arachnoid mater
- Arachnoid mater (cut and reflected)
- Meninges: Pia mater
- Arachnoid mater
- Dura mater

- Superior sagittal sinus
- Arachnoid granulations
- Periosteal layer of dura mater removed to show superior sagittal sinus
- Openings of superior cerebral veins draining into superior sagittal sinus
- Lateral lacuna
- Meningeal branch of anterior ethmoidal artery
- Middle meningeal vein and artery

What to look for

Symptoms can occur very suddenly.

- Fever
- Headache
- Neck pain or stiffness
- Nausea and vomiting
- Fatigue
- Rash and petechiae
- Flu-like symptoms
- Photophobia (sensitivity to light)
- Nuchal rigidity
- Lower back pain
- Positive Brudzinski sign (see image A below)
- Positive Kernig sign (see image B below)
- Seizure
- Motor weakness

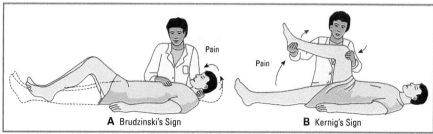

Pain

Pain

A Brudzinski's Sign　　　　　　　**B** Kernig's Sign

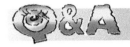

Matchmaker

Match the whiplash injury with its correct name.

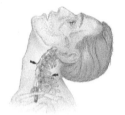 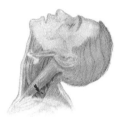 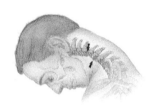

1. _____   2. _____   3. _____

A. muscle injury

B. hyperflexion

C. hyperextension

Able to label?

In the illustration, label the brain structures.

1. _____
2. _____
3. _____
4. _____
5. _____
6. _____
7. _____

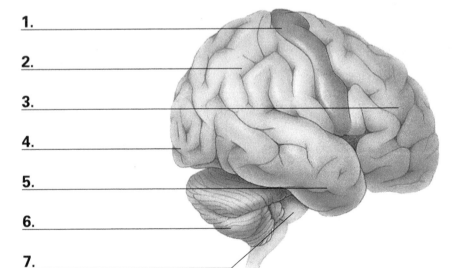

Answers: Matchmaker 1. C, 2. A, 3. B Able to label? 1. motor cortex, 2. parietal lobe, 3. frontal lobe, 4. occipital lobe, 5. temporal lobe, 6. cerebellum, 7. midbrain.

Suggested References

Andersen, H. S., & Hoffman, M. (2015). Alzheimer's disease. Retrieved from: http://emedicine.medscape.com/article/1134817-overview on July 20, 2015.

Bamberger, D. M. (2010). Diagnosis, initial management, and prevention of meningitis. *American Family Physician, 82*(12), 1491–1498.

Centers for Disease Control and Prevention. (2015). Meningitis. Retrieved from: www.cdc.gov/meningitis/index.html on June 13, 2015.

Chawla, J., & Lutsep, H. L. (2015). Migraine headache. Retrieved from: http://emedicine.medscape.com/article/1142556-overview on July 20, 2015.

Cohen-Gadol, A. A., & Bohnstedt, B. N. (2013). Recognition and evaluation of nontraumatic subarachnoid hemorrhage and ruptured cerebral aneurysm. *American Family Physician, 88*(7), 451–456.

Gazewood, J. D., Richards, D. R., & Clebak, K. (2013). Parkinson disease: An update. *American Family Physician, 87*(4), 267–273.

Hunter, O. K., & Lorenzo, C. T. (2015). Cervical strain and sprain. Retrieved from: http://emedicine.medscape.com/article/306176-overview on July 17, 2015.

Kumar, V., Abbas, A., & Aster, J. (2015). *Robbins & Cotran pathologic basis of disease.* Philadelphia, PA: Elsevier-Saunders.

Manning, J. S. (2015). Practical approaches in the management of bipolar depression: Overcoming challenges and avoiding pitfalls. Bipolar disorder, bipolar depression and comorbid illness. *Journal of Family Practice, 64*(6 suppl), S10–S15.

Nicholas, R., & Rashid, W. (2013). Multiple sclerosis. *American Family Physician, 87*(10), 712–714.

Posner, E. (2015). Absence seizures in children. *American Family Physician, 91*(2), 114–115.

Russell, G., & Nicol, P. (2009). "I've broken my neck or something!" The general practice experience of whiplash. *Family Practice, 26*(2), 115–120.

Saguil, A., Kane, S., & Farnell, E. (2014). Multiple sclerosis: A primary care perspective. *American Family Physician, 90*(9), 644–652.

Shah, A., & Lorenzo, N. (2015). Myasthenia gravis. Retrieved from: http://emedicine.medscape.com/article/1171206-overview on July 19, 2015.

Wilden, J. A., & Cohen-Gadol, A. A. (2012). Evaluation of first nonfebrile seizures. *American Family Physician, 86*(4), 334–340.

Yancey, J. R., Sheridan, R., & Koren, K. G. (2014). Chronic daily headache: Diagnosis and management. *American Family Physician, 89*(8), 642–648.

Yew, K. S., & Cheng, E. M. (2015). Diagnosis of acute stroke. *American Family Physician, 91*(8), 528–536.

Gastrointestinal disorders

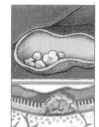
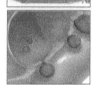
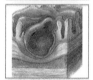
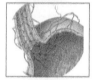

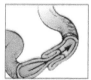
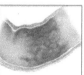
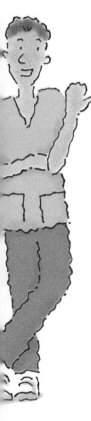

Cholecystitis

Gastrointestinal

In cholecystitis, the gallbladder becomes inflamed. Usually, a calculus (gallstone) becomes lodged in the cystic duct, causing painful gallbladder distention. Cholecystitis may be acute or chronic.

Understanding gallstone formation

Abnormal metabolism of cholesterol and bile salts plays an important role in gallstone formation. The liver makes bile continuously. The gallbladder concentrates and stores it until the duodenum signals it needs bile to help digest fat. Changes in the composition of bile may allow gallstones to form. Changes to the absorptive ability of the gallbladder lining may also contribute to gallstone formation.

> Cholesterol metabolism and bile salts seem to be the main culprits at this point.

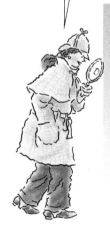

How it happens

Cholecystitis results from the formation of gallstones. The exact cause of gallstone formation is unknown, but it's thought that abnormal metabolism of cholesterol and bile salts plays an important role. Acute cholecystitis may also be due to poor or absent blood flow to the gallbladder.

1 Inside the liver

Certain conditions, such as age, obesity, and estrogen imbalance, cause the liver to secrete bile that's abnormally high in cholesterol or lacking the proper concentration of bile salts.

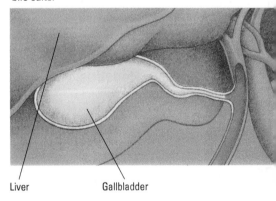

Liver   Gallbladder

2 Inside the gallbladder

When the gallbladder concentrates bile, inflammation may occur. Excessive reabsorption of water and bile salts makes the bile less soluble. Cholesterol, calcium, and bilirubin precipitate into gallstones.

Fat entering the duodenum causes the intestinal mucosa to secrete the hormone cholecystokinin, which stimulates the gallbladder to contract and empty. If a stone lodges in the cystic duct, the gallbladder contracts but can't empty, resulting in inflammation and pain.

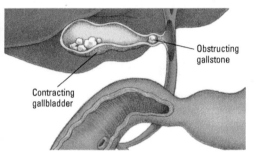

Obstructing gallstone

Contracting gallbladder

age-old story

Age and cholecystitis

The acute form of cholecystitis is most common during middle age; the chronic form occurs most often in elderly people. Children with sickle cell disease, severe illness, or congenital or biliary anomalies and those on prolonged total parenteral nutrition may present without the typical symptoms.

4 Inside the biliary tree

Inflammation can progress up the biliary tree into any of the bile ducts. This can cause pancreatitis.

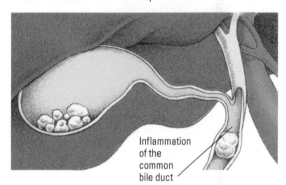

Inflammation of the common bile duct

3 Inside the common bile duct

If a stone lodges in the common bile duct, the bile can't flow into the duodenum. When bile is unable to flow freely from the liver, bilirubin backs up into the blood and causes jaundice.

Biliary duct spasm and swelling of the tissue around the stone can also cause irritation and inflammation of the common bile duct. The biliary duct spasm causes waves of pain called biliary colic.

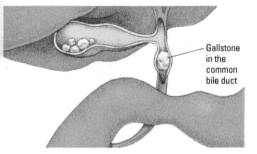

Gallstone in the common bile duct

What to look for

- Acute abdominal pain in the right upper quadrant that may radiate to the back, between the shoulders, or to the front of the chest (in the elderly, symptoms are often vague and may progress rapidly)
- Colic type pain in the right upper quadrant of the abdomen (waves of steady cramping pain)
- Nausea and vomiting
- Jaundice
- Belching
- Flatulence
- Indigestion

Cirrhosis

Cirrhosis, a manifestation of chronic liver disease, is characterized by widespread destruction of hepatic cells, which are replaced by fibrous cells through a process called *fibrotic regeneration*.

How it happens

The changes that occur in cirrhosis, such as irreversible chronic injury of the liver, extensive fibrosis, and nodular tissue growth, result from liver cell death, collapse of the liver's supporting structure, distortion of the vascular bed, and nodular regeneration of remaining liver tissue.

Many causes of chronic liver injury can lead to cirrhosis. The two most common causes of chronic liver injury in the United States are alcoholic liver disease and hepatitis C. Other causes include

- primary biliary cirrhosis
- primary sclerosing cholangitis
- autoimmune hepatitis
- chronic hepatitis B
- hereditary hemochromatosis
- Wilson disease
- alpha-1 antitrypsin deficiency
- nonalcoholic fatty liver disease

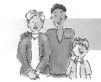

age-old story

Age and cirrhosis

Cirrhosis is especially prevalent among people older than age 50 with chronic alcoholism; it's also twice as common in men as in women.

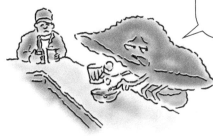

Alcohol is not a friend, especially if the person is male and middle-aged.

Malnutrition also plays a role in cirrhosis. This spread would have done a cirrhosis patient some good! Thiamine supplements are particularly needed.

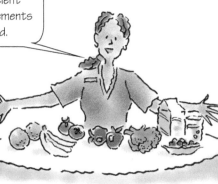

Cirrhosis of the liver

The surface of the liver shows small nodules as opposed to the normally smooth surface.

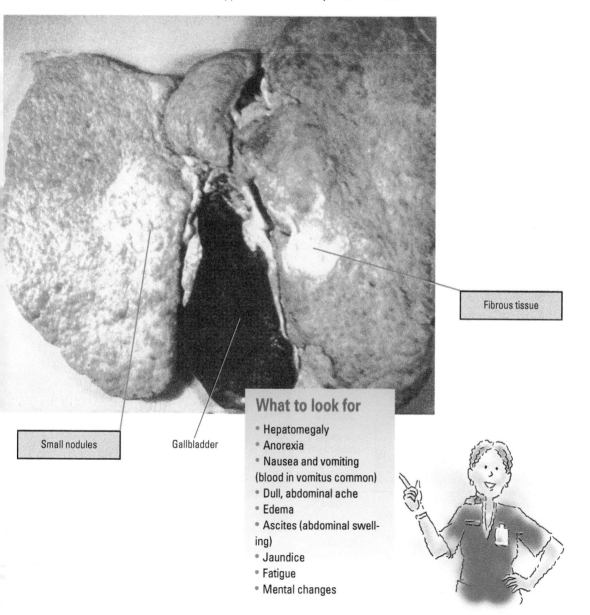

Fibrous tissue

Small nodules

Gallbladder

What to look for

- Hepatomegaly
- Anorexia
- Nausea and vomiting (blood in vomitus common)
- Dull, abdominal ache
- Edema
- Ascites (abdominal swelling)
- Jaundice
- Fatigue
- Mental changes

Colorectal cancer

Colorectal cancer is a slow-growing adenocarcinoma that usually starts in the inner layer of the intestinal tract. It commonly begins as a polyp and is potentially curable if diagnosed early.

Types of colorectal cancer

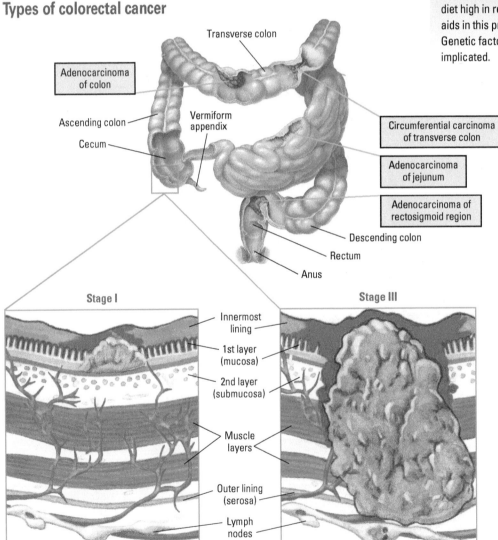

Age and colorectal cancer

Being older than age 40 is a risk factor for colorectal cancer.

What to look for

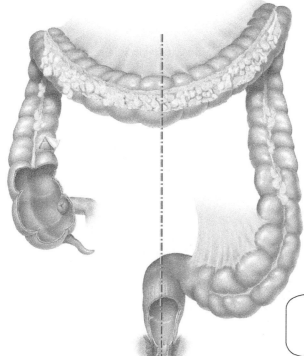

On the right

- Black, tarry stools
- Rectal bleeding
- Anemia
- Abdominal aching, pressure, or dull cramps
- Weakness
- Fatigue
- Exertional dyspnea
- Diarrhea
- Obstipation
- Anorexia
- Weight loss
- Vomiting
- Change in caliber of stool

On the left

- Black, tarry stools or rectal bleeding
- Intermittent abdominal fullness or cramping; rectal pressure
- Obstipation
- Diarrhea or "ribbonlike" stool
- Dark or bright red blood in stool; mucus in or on stool

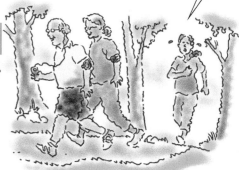

I'm glad all I inherited was my love of jogging. How much farther?

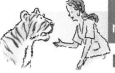

risky business

Risk factors for colorectal cancer

- Inherited gene mutations
- Family or personal history of colorectal cancer, Crohn disease, or ulcerative colitis
- History of intestinal polyps
- Aging
- High-fat diet
- Obesity and physical inactivity
- Diabetes
- Smoking
- Heavy alcohol intake

Crohn disease

Crohn disease is one of two major types of inflammatory bowel disease (IBD). It may affect any part of the gastrointestinal (GI) tract although it is most common in the small intestine and the beginning of the large intestine. Inflammation extends through all layers of the intestinal wall and may involve lymph nodes and supporting membranes. Ulcers form as the inflammation extends into the peritoneum. Crohn disease is prevalent in adults aged 20 to 40; however, it is most prevalent in those aged 20 to 29.

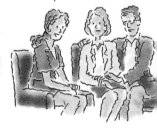

Crohn disease affects men and women equally. It also tends to run in families—up to 20% of patients with the disease have a history of it in their family.

How it happens

I'm not quite sure I want to play…

Start

1 Lymph nodes enlarge, and lymph flow into the submucosa is blocked.

2 Lymphatic obstruction causes edema, mucosal ulceration, fissures, abscesses, and, sometimes, granulomas. Mucosal ulcerations are called *skipping lesions* because they aren't continuous (as in ulcerative colitis).

Skipping Lesions

3 Oval, elevated patches of closely packed lymph follicles on the lining of the small intestine—called *Peyer patches*—become inflamed.

Peyer's Patches

End

6 Eventually, diseased parts of the bowel become thicker, narrower, and shorter and can lead to formation of strictures.

5 Inflammation of the serous membrane (serositis) develops, inflamed bowel loops adhere to other diseased or normal loops, and diseased bowel segments become interspersed with healthy ones.

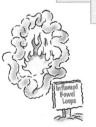

Inflamed Bowel Loops

4 Fibrosis occurs, thickening the bowel wall and causing stenosis, or narrowing of the lumen.

A closer look

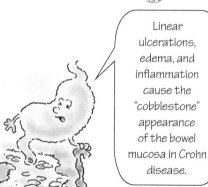

Serosa
Muscularis
Uninvolved (skipped) area

Narrow lumen
Thickened wall
Linear ulceration
Hyperplastic lymph node
Granuloma
Lymphoid follicle
Perforation
Abscess

Fistula into loop of small bowel

Granulomatous lymphadenitis
Transmural chronic inflammation

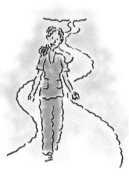

Mucosal surface of the bowel in Crohn disease

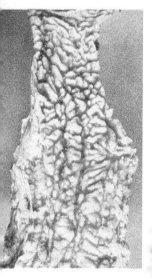

Linear ulcerations, edema, and inflammation cause the "cobblestone" appearance of the bowel mucosa in Crohn disease.

What to look for

- Malaise
- Diarrhea (bloody diarrhea is common)
- Pain in the right lower quadrant
- Generalized abdominal cramping/pain
- Fever
- Weight loss
- Anemia
- Fatigue
- Nausea
- Loss of appetite

Diverticular disease

In diverticular disease, bulging, pouchlike herniations (diverticula) in the GI wall push the mucosal lining through the surrounding muscle. Diverticula occur most commonly in the sigmoid colon, but they may develop anywhere, from the proximal end of the pharynx to the anus.

Diverticular disease has two clinical forms:

1 Diverticulosis—diverticula are present but produce no symptoms.

2 Diverticulitis—inflamed diverticula that may cause potentially fatal obstruction, infection, and hemorrhage.

> Location is everything in real estate. Diverticular disease can occur anywhere along the digestive tract, but it's most common on the left side of the colon.

How it happens

Diverticula probably result from high intraluminal pressure on an area of weakness in the GI wall where blood vessels enter. Diet may be a contributing factor because insufficient fiber reduces fecal residue, narrows the bowel lumen, and leads to high intra-abdominal pressure during defecation.

In diverticulitis, retained undigested food and bacteria accumulate in the diverticular sac. This hard mass cuts off the blood supply to the thin walls of the sac, making them more susceptible to attack by colonic bacteria. Inflammation follows and may lead to perforation, abscess, peritonitis, obstruction, or hemorrhage. Occasionally, the inflamed colon segment may adhere to the bladder or other organs and cause a fistula.

age-old story

Age and diverticular disease

Diverticular disease is most prevalent in men older than age 40 and in people who eat a low-fiber diet. More than one-half of all people older than age 50 have colonic diverticula.

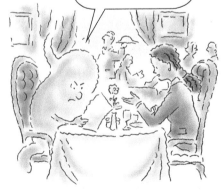

> I hate having to watch my diet because of this diverticulitis. I tell you, it isn't fair!

Diverticulosis of the colon

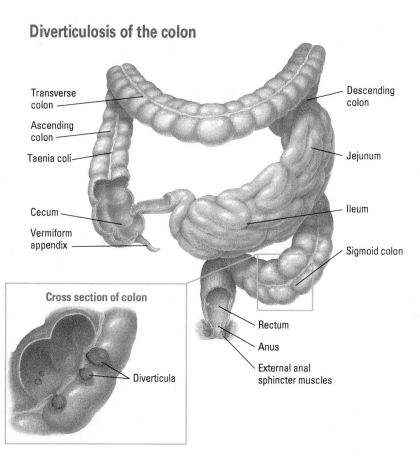

Transverse colon

Ascending colon

Taenia coli

Cecum

Vermiform appendix

Descending colon

Jejunum

Ileum

Sigmoid colon

Rectum

Anus

External anal sphincter muscles

Cross section of colon

Diverticula

What to look for

Typically, the patient with diverticulosis is asymptomatic and will remain so unless diverticulitis develops.

Mild
* Moderate left-sided lower abdominal pain in 70% of patients
* Low-grade fever
* Change in bowel habits

Severe
* Abdominal rigidity
* Left lower quadrant pain
* High fever
* Chills
* Hypotension

Chronic
* Constipation
* Ribbonlike stools
* Intermittent diarrhea
* Abdominal distention
* Abdominal rigidity and pain
* Diminishing or absent bowel sounds
* Nausea
* Vomiting

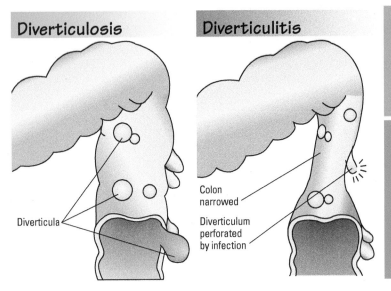

Diverticulosis

Diverticulitis

Diverticula

Colon narrowed

Diverticulum perforated by infection

Peptic ulcer disease

Peptic ulcer disease is a disorder of inflammation and ulceration of the duodenum or stomach. It is most often due to a bacterial infection or over use of nonsteroidal anti-inflammatory drug (NSAID)-type medication (such as aspirin or ibuprofen). The bacteria is called *Helicobacter pylori,* and it has the ability to invade submucosal areas of the duodenum and stomach and secrete an enzyme that causes inflammation and protects the organism from acid. Alternatively, NSAID medications diminish the gastric mucus that protects the lining of the stomach, and then acid can irritate and ulcerate the membranes.

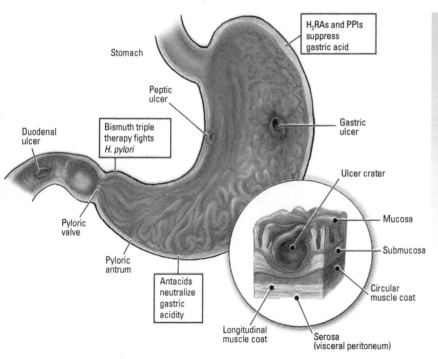

H₂RAs and PPIs suppress gastric acid

Stomach

Peptic ulcer

Duodenal ulcer

Bismuth triple therapy fights *H. pylori*

Gastric ulcer

Ulcer crater

Pyloric valve

Pyloric antrum

Antacids neutralize gastric acidity

Mucosa

Submucosa

Circular muscle coat

Longitudinal muscle coat

Serosa (visceral peritoneum)

What to look for

* Burning, gnawing epigastric pain (especially between meals)
* Acid reflux causing bitter taste in mouth
* Frequent heartburn
* Belching
* Bloated feeling
* Anorexia
* Nausea
* Possible dark stool (due to blood in stool)
* Epigastric pain radiating to the back can indicate penetrating peptic ulcer (emergency)

Esophageal varices

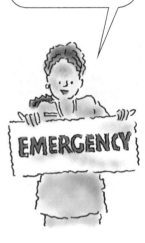

Esophageal varices can require emergency care if massive hemorrhage occurs.

Esophageal varices are dilated tortuous veins in the submucosa of the lower esophagus. In many patients, they're the first sign of portal hypertension (elevated pressure in the portal vein due to liver disease). Esophageal varices commonly cause massive hematemesis (vomiting of blood), requiring emergency care to control hemorrhage and prevent hypovolemic shock.

How it happens

Portal hypertension occurs when blood meets increased resistance in the liver commonly due to a chronic hepatic disorder. As pressure in the portal vein increases, blood backs up into the spleen, stomach, and lower esophagus. The backed-up blood causes dilated, distended fragile veins. Around the lower esophagus, the distended veins are called esophageal varices, and they easily rupture and can cause hemorrhage.

I get totally passed by when portal hypertension occurs. Bad news for the esophagus.

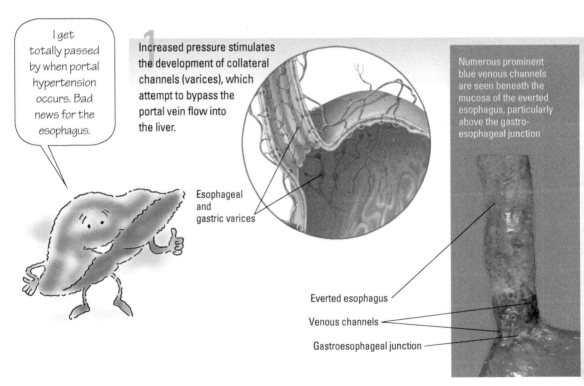

1 Increased pressure stimulates the development of collateral channels (varices), which attempt to bypass the portal vein flow into the liver.

Esophageal and gastric varices

Numerous prominent blue venous channels are seen beneath the mucosa of the everted esophagus, particularly above the gastro-esophageal junction

Everted esophagus

Venous channels

Gastroesophageal junction

What happens in portal hypertension

Portal hypertension (elevated pressure in the portal vein) occurs when blood flow meets increased resistance, which most commonly occurs in cirrhosis of the liver.

As the pressure in the portal vein rises, blood backs up into the spleen and flows through collateral channels to the venous system, bypassing the liver. Thus, portal hypertension causes
• splenomegaly
• dilated collateral veins (esophageal varices, hemorrhoids, or prominent abdominal veins)
• ascites

In many patients, the first sign of portal hypertension is bleeding esophageal varices (dilated tortuous veins in the submucosa of the lower esophagus).

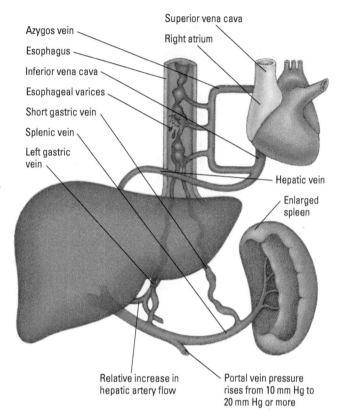

As pressure in the portal vein rises, blood backs up into the spleen.

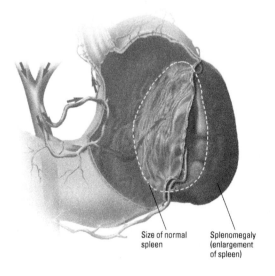

What to look for

• Weakness, fatigue, malaise
• Anorexia, weight loss
• Hypotension
• Cyanosis of the lips, tongue, and periphery
• Altered level of consciousness
• Hematemesis (bloody vomitus; sometimes called "coffee ground" emesis)
• Dyspnea
• Tachycardia

Gastroesophageal reflux disease

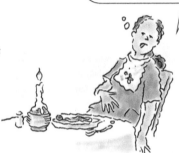

I probably shouldn't have had that extra helping of pasta. The sauce was pretty garlicky...

Popularly known as *heartburn*, gastroesophageal reflux disease (GERD) refers to the excess backflow of gastric and duodenal contents past the lower esophageal sphincter (LES) and into the esophagus without associated belching or vomiting. The reflux of gastric contents causes acute epigastric pain, usually after a meal. The pain may radiate to the chest or arms.

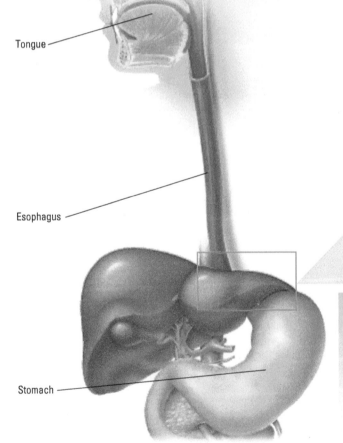

Tongue

Esophagus

Stomach

What to look for

- Burning pain in the epigastric area, possibly radiating to the arms and chest
- Pain, usually after a meal or when lying down
- Feeling of fluid accumulation in the throat with a sour or bitter taste
- Coughing
- Sore throat, hoarseness
- Dysphagia

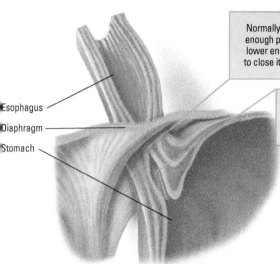

Normally, the LES maintains enough pressure around the lower end of the esophagus to close it and prevent reflux.

Typically, the sphincter relaxes after each swallow to allow food into the stomach.

Esophagus

Diaphragm

Stomach

Want a sour taste? Suck on a lemon. Or, think about what it feels like to have GERD.

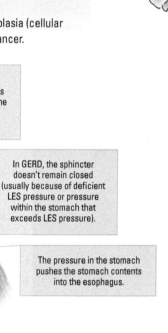

How it happens

1. The high acidity of the stomach contents causes irritation of the lower esophageal sphincter, a muscle that closes off the esophagus from the stomach.
2. In GERD, the lower esophageal sphincter doesn't completely close.
3. The lack of closure of the sphincter allows gastric acid contents to reflux up and irritate the lower esophageal epithelium, causing inflammation.
4. With repeated episodes of reflux of acid, GERD can lead to metaplasia (cellular change) of the lower esophagus and susceptibility to esophageal cancer.

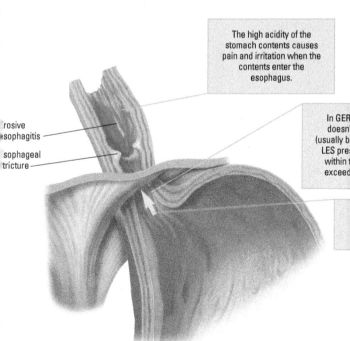

The high acidity of the stomach contents causes pain and irritation when the contents enter the esophagus.

In GERD, the sphincter doesn't remain closed (usually because of deficient LES pressure or pressure within the stomach that exceeds LES pressure).

The pressure in the stomach pushes the stomach contents into the esophagus.

Erosive esophagitis

Esophageal stricture

Hepatitis, viral

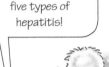

We're the five types of hepatitis!

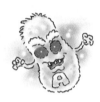
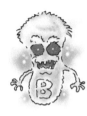
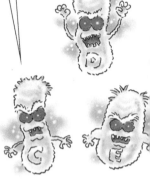

Viral hepatitis is a common infection of the liver. There are 5 kinds of viruses: hepatitis A, B, C, D, and E. Most common viral causes in the United States are hepatitis A virus (HAV), hepatitis B virus (HBV), and hepatitis C virus (HCV). Hepatitis A causes a severe gastroenteritis-like infection usually from contaminated food. HAV causes no permanent damage, and full recovery is expected. However, Hepatitis B and hepatitis C can cause more prolonged liver dysfunction and chronic illness. There is a vaccine and treatment for hepatitis B. However, there is no vaccine for hepatitis C, and treatment is more challenging.

How it happens

The virus causes hepatocyte injury and death, either by directly killing the cells or by activating inflammatory and immune reactions. The inflammatory and immune reactions, in turn, injure or destroy hepatocytes by causing the infected or neighboring cells to disintegrate. Later, direct antibody attack against the viral antigens causes further destruction of the infected cells. Edema and swelling of the liver interstitium lead to collapse of capillaries, decreased blood flow, tissue hypoxia, scarring, and fibrosis.

In the adult population, acute hepatitis A is symptomatic and treatable, while acute hepatitis B or C may be asymptomatic.

Approximately 1% of patients with acute hepatitis due to hepatitis B or C develop fulminant hepatic failure (FHF) and can develop liver cancer.

Liver with the effects of hepatitis

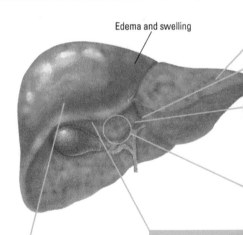

Edema and swelling

Hepatitis B

Blood-borne—parenteral route, sexual, maternal neonatal; virus is shed in all body fluids

Hepatitis A

Highly contagious; results from ingestion of contaminated food or water

Normal liver

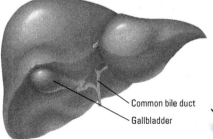

Common bile duct

Gallbladder

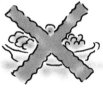

Hepatitis E

Associated with recent travel to endemic areas such as India, Africa, Asia, or Central America; fecal-oral route

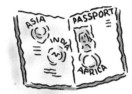

Hepatitis D

Linked to chronic hepatitis B infection

Hepatitis C

Blood-borne: parenteral route associated with shared needles, blood transfusions, but it can also be transmitted sexually or by mother to her fetus

What to look for

Prodromal stage
- Fatigue
- Anorexia
- Dyspepsia
- Malaise
- Arthralgia
- Myalgia
- Fever
- Mild weight loss
- Nausea and vomiting
- Changes in senses of taste and smell
- Right upper quadrant tenderness
- Dark-colored urine
- Clay-colored stools

Clinical or icteric stage
- Itching
- Jaundice
- Abdominal pain or tenderness
- High aminotransferase (liver enzyme) values
- Hyperbilirubinemia

Recovery stage
- Subsiding symptoms
- Return of appetite

Moderate hepatitis

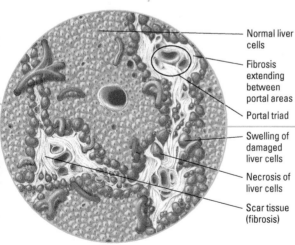

- Normal liver cells
- Fibrosis extending between portal areas
- Portal triad
- Swelling of damaged liver cells
- Necrosis of liver cells
- Scar tissue (fibrosis)

Necrotic liver

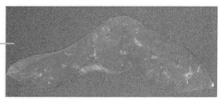

A necrotic liver becomes soft and smaller in size than a normal liver.

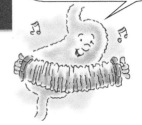

A bowel free from obstruction is music to my ears!

Intestinal obstruction

Intestinal obstruction is the partial or complete blockage of the lumen in the small or large bowel. Small bowel obstruction is far more common and usually more serious. Complete obstruction in any part of the small or large bowel, if untreated, can cause death within hours due to shock and vascular collapse. Intestinal obstruction is most likely to occur after abdominal surgery or in persons with congenital bowel deformities. Sixty percent of small bowel obstructions (SBO) in the United States are caused by postoperative adhesions.

Obstruction in the small intestine results in metabolic alkalosis from dehydration and loss of gastric hydrochloric acid; lower bowel obstruction causes slower dehydration and loss of intestinal alkaline fluids, resulting in metabolic acidosis. Ultimately, intestinal obstruction may lead to ischemia, necrosis, and death.

Intestinal obstruction develops in three forms.

Simple—Blockage prevents intestinal contents from passing, with no other complications.	*Strangulated*—In addition to blockage of the lumen, blood supply to part or all of the obstructed section is cut off.	*Close-looped*—Both ends of a bowel section are occluded, isolating it from the rest of the intestine.

How it happens

The physiologic effects are similar in all three forms of obstruction. When intestinal obstruction occurs, fluid, air, and gas collect near the obstruction. Pain builds in the abdomen. The abdomen becomes tender and rigid. Peristalsis increases temporarily as the bowel tries to force its contents through the obstruction, injuring intestinal mucosa and causing distention at and above the site of the obstruction. Distention blocks the flow of venous blood and halts normal absorptive processes; as a result, the bowel wall becomes edematous and begins to secrete water, sodium, and potassium into the fluid pooled in the lumen.

Three causes of intestinal obstruction

1. Intussusception with invagination or shortening of the bowel caused by the involution of one segment of the bowel into another.

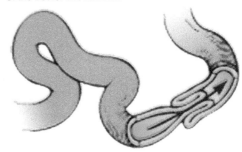

2. Volvulus of the sigmoid colon; the twist is counterclockwise in most cases.

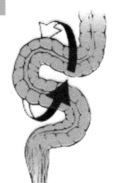

3. Hernia (inguinal): the sac of the hernia is a continuation of the peritoneum of the abdomen. The hernial contents are the intestine, omentum, or other abdominal contents that pass through the hernial opening into the hernial sac.

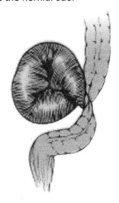

Age and intestinal obstruction

Intussusception, or the telescoping of the bowel into another segment, is the most common cause of intestinal obstruction in children younger than age 2. Colonic obstruction is more prevalent among the elderly and may be associated with malignancy.

What to look for

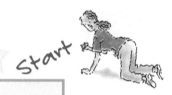

Start

> If you suspect I have intestinal obstruction, it's probably intussusception. Boy, that's a long word!

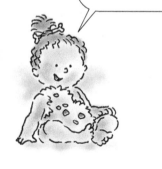

Obstruction

Fluid, gas, and air collect behind obstruction.

Peristalsis temporarily increases in attempt to force contents past obstruction.

Distention increases at and above obstruction site.

Distention impedes blood supply to the bowel, halting absorption.

Bowel wall swells as water, sodium, and potassium are secreted into intestine and not absorbed from it.

Gas-forming bacteria collect above obstruction, increasing distention.

Dehydration results because fluids aren't absorbed into the bloodstream.

With no treatment, severe hypovolemia occurs.

Gas-forming bacteria collect above the obstruction, increasing distention.

Sepsis

Death

Ulcerative colitis

Ulcerative colitis is an inflammatory disease that affects the mucosa of the colon and rectum. It invariably begins in the rectum and sigmoid colon, rarely affecting the small intestine, except for the terminal ileum in about 10% of cases and due to an incompetent ileocecal valve. Ulcerative colitis produces edema (leading to mucosal friability) and ulcerations. The disease cycles between exacerbation and remission. It damages the large intestine's mucosal and submucosal layers.

age-old story

Age and ulcerative colitis

Ulcerative colitis occurs primarily in young adults. Onset of symptoms seems to occur most commonly between ages 15 and 30 and between ages 55 and 65.

How it happens

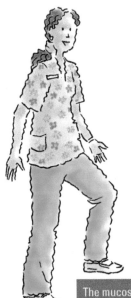

> Ch-ch-changes...I used to have a normal colon attached, but with the progression of ulcerative colitis, my buddy the colon has gone through some changes...

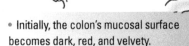

Usually, the disease originates in the rectum (95% of the time) and lower colon. Then it spreads to the entire colon.

The mucosa develops diffuse ulceration, with hemorrhage, congestion, edema, and exudative inflammation. Ulcerations are continuous (unlike Crohn disease, which has skipped areas)

Abscesses formed in the mucosa drain purulent pus, become necrotic, and ulcerate.

Sloughing occurs, causing bloody, mucus-filled stools.

- Initially, the colon's mucosal surface becomes dark, red, and velvety.
- Abscesses form and coalesce into ulcers.
- Necrosis of the mucosa occurs.
- As abscesses heal, scarring and thickening may appear in the bowel's inner muscle layer.
- As granulation tissue replaces the muscle layer, the colon narrows, shortens, and loses its characteristic pouches (haustral folds).

Mucosal changes in ulcerative colitis

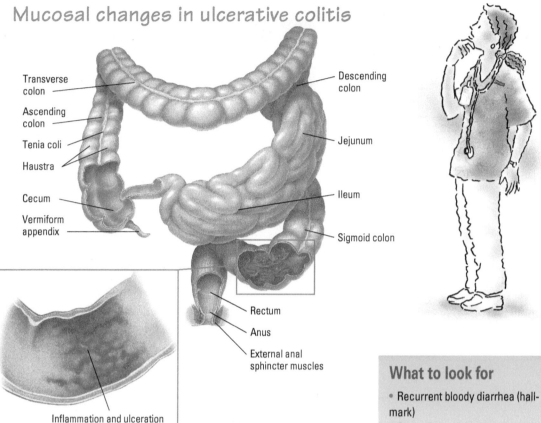

Transverse colon

Ascending colon

Tenia coli

Haustra

Cecum

Vermiform appendix

Descending colon

Jejunum

Ileum

Sigmoid colon

Rectum

Anus

External anal sphincter muscles

Inflammation and ulceration

Colon with ulcerative colitis

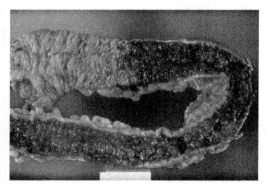

Prominent erythema and ulceration of the colon begin in the ascending colon and are most severe in the rectosigmoid area.

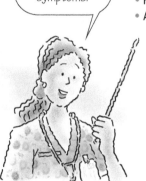

Pay attention to these telling signs and symptoms.

What to look for

- Recurrent bloody diarrhea (hallmark)
- Cramping, pain, rectal urgency, and diarrhea (from accumulation of blood and mucus in the bowel)
- Weight loss
- Anorexia
- Nausea
- Vomiting
- Weakness
- Fever
- Abdominal distention

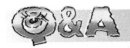

Show and tell
Name the two types of diverticular disease shown at the right and then define them.

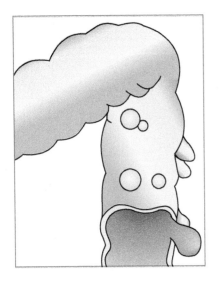

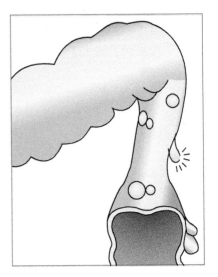

1. _____

_____

2. _____

_____

Riddle
Solve the riddle to find out a way to help avoid many GI disorders, including colorectal cancer.

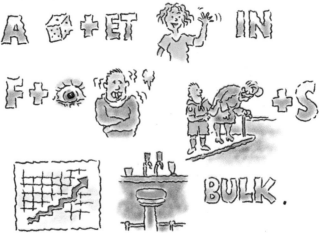

Selected References

Cholecystitis

Bloom, A. (2014). Cholecystitis: Clinical Presentation. Retrieved from: http://emedicine.medscape.com/article/171886-clinical on June 19, 2015.

Ilige, M., Meyer, A., & Kovach, F. (2014). Surgical treatment for asymptomatic cholelithiasis. *American Family Physician, 89*(6), 468–470.

Cirrhosis

Starr, S. P., & Raines, D. (2011). Cirrhosis: Diagnosis, management, and prevention. *American Family Physician, 84*(12), 1353–1359.

Wolf, D. (2014). Cirrhosis: Practice essentials, overview, epidemiology. Retrieved from: http://emedicine.medscape.com/article/185856 on June 19, 2015.

Colon Cancer

Brenner, H., Kloor, M., & Pox, C. P. (2014). Colorectal cancer. *Lancet, 383*(9927), 1490–1502.

Dragovich, T. (2015). Colon cancer. Retrieved from: http://emedicine.medscape.com/article/277496 on June 19, 2015.

Crohn Disease

Molodecky, N. A., Soon, I. S., Rabi, D. M., Ghali, W. A., Ferris, M., Chernoff, G., ... Kaplan, G. G. (2012). Increasing incidence and prevalence of the inflammatory bowel diseases with time, based on systematic review. *Gastroenterology, 142*(1), 46–54.

NIH. (2014). Crohn's disease. NIH Publication No. 14–3410. Retrieved from: http://www.niddk.nih.gov/health-information/health-topics/digestive-diseases/crohns-disease/Pages/facts.aspx on July 18, 2015.

Wilkins, T., Jarvis, K., & Patel, J. (2011). Diagnosis and management of Crohn's disease. *American Family Physician, 84*(12), 1365–1375.

Diverticulosis/Diverticulitis

Cunha, J. (2015). Diverticulitis vs. diverticulosis. Retrieved from: http://www.emedicinehealth.com/diverticulosis_and_diverticulitis/page2_em.htm#diverticulitis_vs_diverticulosis on July 18, 2015.

Humes, D., Smith, J. K., & Spiller, R. C. (2011). Colonic diverticular disease. *American Family Physician, 84*(10), 1163–1164.

Shahedi, K. (2015). Diverticulitis. Retrieved from: http://emedicine.medscape.com/article/173388 on July 18, 2015.

Esophageal Varices

Carale, J. (2014). Portal hypertension. Retrieved from: http://emedicine.medscape.com/article/182098 on July 18, 2015.

LeBreche, D. (2013). Esophageal varices. Retrieved from: http://www.worldgastroenterology.org/assets/export/userfiles/2014_FINAL_ESOPHAGEAL-VARICES.pdf on July 18, 2015.

Wilkins, T., Khan, N., Nabh, A., & Schade, R. R. (2012). Diagnosis and management of upper gastrointestinal bleeding. *American Family Physician, 85*(5), 469–476.

Gastroesophageal Reflux Disease

Patti, M. (2014). Gastroesophageal reflux disease. Retrieved from: http://emedicine.medscape.com/article/176595 on July 18, 2015.

Leehusen, D. A., & Escano, J. (2012). Managing chronic gastroesophageal reflux disease. *American Family Physician, 86*(7), 617–619.

Hepatitis, Viral

Buggs, A. M. (2014). Viral hepatitis. Retrieved from: http://emedicine.medscape.com/article/775507 on July 18, 2015.

Matheny, S. C., & Kingery, J. E. (2012). Hepatitis A. *American Family Physician, 86*(11), 1027–1034.

Wilkins, T., Akhtar, M., Gititu, E., Jalluri, C., & Ramirez, J. (2015). Diagnosis and management of hepatitis C. *American Family Physician, 91*(12), 835–842.

Intestinal Obstruction

Hopkins, C. (2014). Large-bowel obstruction. Retrieved from: http://emedicine.medscape.com/article/774045 on July 18, 2015.

Jackson, P. G., & Raiji, M. T. (2011). Evaluation and management of intestinal obstruction. *American Family Physician, 83*(2), 159–165.

Nobie, B. A. Small-bowel obstruction. Retrieved from: http://emedicine.medscape.com/article/774140 on July 18, 2015.

Peptic Ulcer

Anand, B. S., & Katz, J. (2015). Peptic ulcer disease. Retrieved from: http://emedicine.medscape.com/article/181753-clinical on July 21, 2015.

Fashner, J., & Gitu, A. C. (2015). Diagnosis and treatment of peptic ulcer disease and *H. pylori* infection. *American Family Physician, 91*(4), 236–242.

Ulcerative Colitis

Adams, S. M., & Bornemann, P. H. (2013). Ulcerative colitis. *American Family Physician, 87*(10), 699–705.

Basson, M. D. (2014). Ulcerative colitis. Retrieved from: http://emedicine.medscape.com/article/183084 on July 18, 2015.

Chapter 6

Musculoskeletal disorders

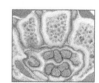

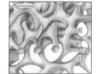
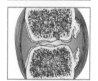
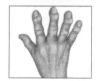
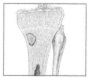
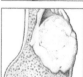
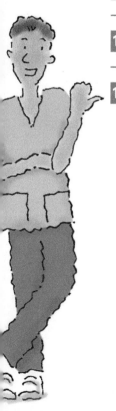

Carpal tunnel syndrome

The most common of the nerve entrapment syndromes, carpal tunnel syndrome (CTS) results from compression of the median nerve at the wrist within the carpal tunnel.

How it happens

The carpal bones and the transverse carpal ligament form the carpal tunnel. Inflammation or fibrosis of the tendon sheaths that pass through the carpal tunnel usually causes edema and compression of the median nerve. This compression neuropathy causes sensory and motor changes in the median nerve distribution of the hands, initially impairing sensory transmission to the thumb, index finger, middle (second) finger, and inner aspect of the ring (fourth) finger. Repetitive or cumulative trauma to the wrist causes CTS.

Continuous or periodic compression on a nerve can cause damage over time. Certain nerves are located in regions of the body that are especially vulnerable to compression injuries. The carpal tunnel is one such region.

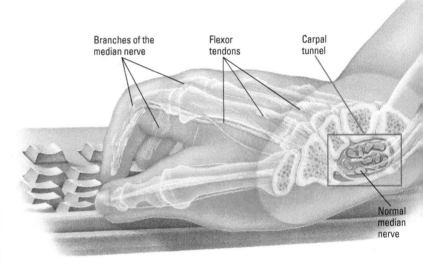

Branches of the median nerve

Flexor tendons

Carpal tunnel

Normal median nerve

Other common causes

Systemic disorders, such as diabetes, rheumatoid arthritis, hypothyroidism, and amyloidosis can be a risk factor.

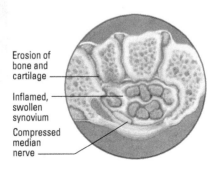

Erosion of bone and cartilage

Inflamed, swollen synovium

Compressed median nerve

Repetitive trauma

Repetitive movements cause cumulative trauma that expose the nerve to compression forces and stretching.

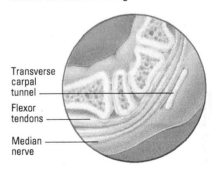

Transverse carpal tunnel

Flexor tendons

Median nerve

Risk factors for carpal tunnel

- Female gender
- Age 40 or older
- Job or hobbies that involve highly repetitive tasks
- Diabetes
- Rheumatoid arthritis

- Hypothyroidism
- Pregnancy
- Trauma to wrist
- Menopause
- Obesity

Cross section of the wrist with CTS

Increased pressure on the median nerve decreases blood flow. If compression persists, the nerve begins to swell. The myelin sheath begins to thin and degenerate.

> One of the main risk factors for carpal tunnel is a job that requires repetitive tasks.

> No bones about it... carpal tunnel syndrome can be very painful.

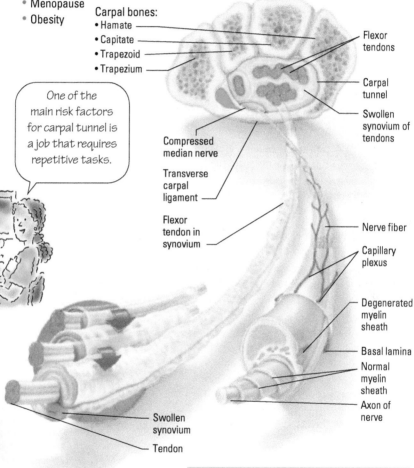

Carpal bones:
- Hamate
- Capitate
- Trapezoid
- Trapezium

Compressed median nerve

Transverse carpal ligament

Flexor tendon in synovium

Flexor tendons

Carpal tunnel

Swollen synovium of tendons

Nerve fiber

Capillary plexus

Degenerated myelin sheath

Basal lamina

Normal myelin sheath

Axon of nerve

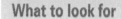

Swollen synovium

Tendon

What to look for

- Weakness, pain, burning, numbness, or tingling in one or both hands
- Paresthesia that affects the thumb, index finger, middle finger, and ring or fourth finger
- Inability to clench the hand into a fist

Herniated disk

A herniated disk, also called a *ruptured* or *slipped disk*, occurs when all or part of the nucleus pulposus—the soft, gelatinous, central portion of the intervertebral disk—protrudes through the disk's weakened or torn outer ring *(annulus fibrosus)*.

age-old story

Age and herniated disks

A herniated disk occurs more frequently in middle-aged and older men. The highest incidence is in the 30- to 50-year age group.

How it happens

An intervertebral disk has two parts: the soft center (nucleus pulposus) and the tough, fibrous surrounding ring (annulus fibrosus). The nucleus pulposus acts as a shock absorber, distributing the mechanical stress applied to the spine when the body moves.

Physical stress, usually a twisting motion, can tear or rupture the annulus fibrosus so that the nucleus pulposus herniates into the spinal canal. The vertebrae move closer together and, in turn, exert pressure on the nerve roots as they exit between the vertebrae. Physical stress, from severe trauma or strain, or intervertebral joint degeneration may cause herniation. Intervertebral disk herniation often causes pain due to sciatic nerve impingement.

"Sciatica" is the pain that radiates from the lower back down the back of the leg. A clinician will check for this by lifting the leg of a supine patient and then dorsiflexing the ankle. If the patient feels back pain, this is called a positive straight leg raising sign, which indicates sciatic nerve impingement.

In older patients whose intervertebral disks have begun to degenerate, even minor trauma may cause herniation.

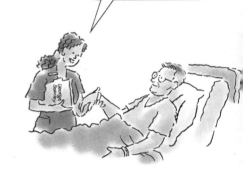

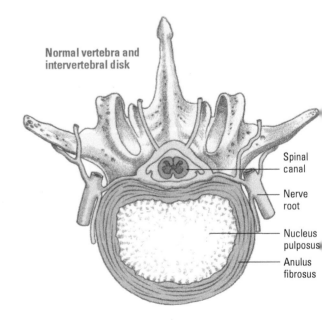

Normal vertebra and intervertebral disk

Spinal canal

Nerve root

Nucleus pulposus

Anulus fibrosus

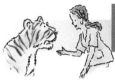

Risk factors for carpal tunnel

- Advancing age
- Male gender
- History of back injury
- Previous herniated disk, or back surgery
- Long periods of sitting, or lifting, or pulling heavy objects
- Frequent bending or twisting of the back
- Heavy physical exertion
- Repetitive motions
- Exposure to constant vibration (such as driving)
- Lack of regular exercise
- Strenuous exercise for a long time, or starting to exercise too strenuously after a long period of inactivity
- Obesity

What to look for

- Severe lower back pain (usually unilateral) that radiates to the buttocks, legs, and feet (called "sciatica")
- Sudden pain after trauma, subsiding after a few days only to return at shorter intervals with progressive intensity
- Sciatic pain after trauma
- Sensory and motor loss in the area innervated by the compressed spinal nerve root
- Difficulty walking on toes or heels
- Weakness and atrophy of leg muscles (later sign)

Protrusion

In protrusion, the nucleus pulposus presses against the annulus fibrosus.

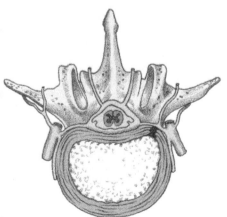

Extrusion and sequestration

In extrusion, the nucleus pulposus bulges forcibly through the annulus fibrosus and impinging on the spinal nerve. Sequestration occurs when the annulus gives way as the disk's core bursts and presses against the nerve root.

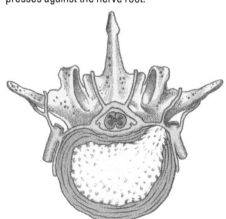

It pains me to say it, but I seem to have a herniated disk!

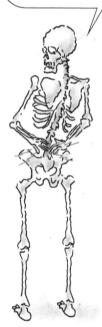

Osteoarthritis

With osteoarthritis, the degree of disability depends on the site of involvement and its severity. I can have minor finger limitation or severe knee disability.

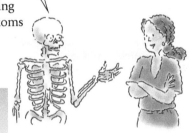

Osteoarthritis, the most common form of arthritis, is widespread, occurring equally in both genders. Symptoms appear after age 40; its earliest symptoms generally begin in middle age and may progress with advancing age.

The rate of progression varies, and joints may remain stable for years in an early stage of deterioration.

How it happens

Osteoarthritis is chronic, causing deterioration of the joint cartilage and formation of reactive new bone called osteophytes at the margins and subchondral (below the cartilage) areas of the joints. This degeneration results from a breakdown of chondrocytes (cartilage cells), most commonly in the hips and knees.

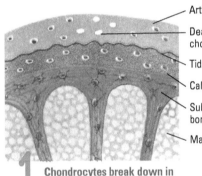

Articular cartilage

Death of chondrocytes

Tide mark

Calcified cartilage

Subchondral bone plate

Marrow

1 Chondrocytes break down in the articular cartilage.

Cloning of chondrocytes

Synovial fluid

Deep crack through tide mark with underlying neovascularization

Osteoblast

Osteoclast

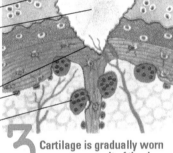

3 Cartilage is gradually worn away as a result of the degeneration of the cartilage and leakage of synovial fluid.

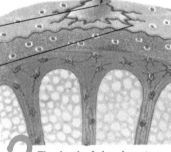

Synovial fluid leaks into crack

Early cracking and fibrillation of cartilage

2 The death of chondrocytes forms a crack in the articular cartilage. Synovial fluid leaks out as the cartilage degenerates.

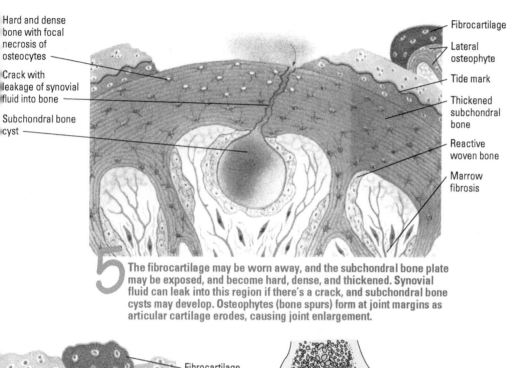

Hard and dense bone with focal necrosis of osteocytes

Crack with leakage of synovial fluid into bone

Subchondral bone cyst

Fibrocartilage

Lateral osteophyte

Tide mark

Thickened subchondral bone

Reactive woven bone

Marrow fibrosis

5 The fibrocartilage may be worn away, and the subchondral bone plate may be exposed, and become hard, dense, and thickened. Synovial fluid can leak into this region if there's a crack, and subchondral bone cysts may develop. Osteophytes (bone spurs) form at joint margins as articular cartilage erodes, causing joint enlargement.

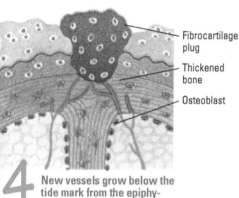

Fibrocartilage plug

Thickened bone

Osteoblast

4 New vessels grow below the tide mark from the epiphysis, and fibrocartilage is formed.

Bone cysts

Osteophyte

Erosion of cartilage and bone

Joint space narrows

6 Joint changes in osteoarthritis

The left side shows early changes and joint space narrowing with cartilage breakdown. The right side shows more severe disease progression with lost cartilage and osteophyte formation.

What to look for

- Deep, aching joint pain, particularly after exercise or weight bearing, that's usually relieved by rest
- Joint stiffness (worse in the morning)
- Aching during changes in weather
- Crepitus (grating) of the joint during motion
- Limited joint movement
- Enlarged distal interphalangeal joints (called Heberden nodes) of the hand
- Enlarged proximal interphalangeal joint (called Bouchard nodes) of the hand

Joints Affected by Osteoarthritis (OA)

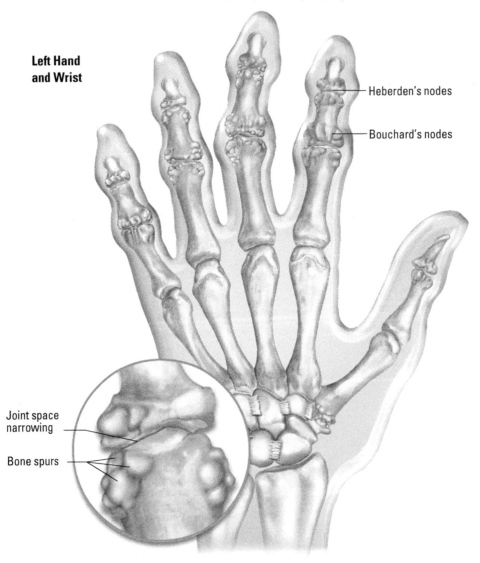

Left Hand and Wrist

Heberden's nodes

Bouchard's nodes

Joint space narrowing

Bone spurs

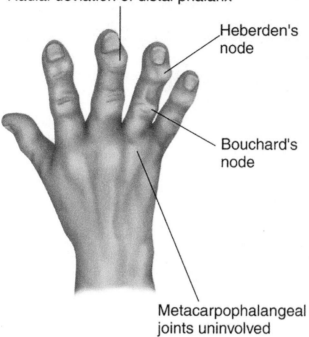

Radial deviation of distal phalanx

Heberden's node

Bouchard's node

Metacarpophalangeal joints uninvolved

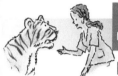

Risk Factors

- OA can be caused by any condition that subjects joint surfaces or underlying bone to chronic, abnormal, or excessive stress; alters articular cartilage in some way; or accelerates the rate of loss of cartilage.

- Trauma, mechanical stress, joint inflammation, medications, or obesity can all contribute to OA.
- Old age is the highest risk for OA of the knee or hip.
- Postmenopausal status is highest risk for OA of the hand.

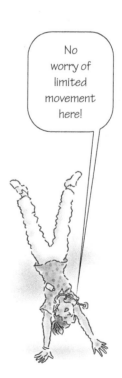

No worry of limited movement here!

Osteomyelitis

Osteomyelitis is a bone infection characterized by a progressive inflammatory reaction that destroys the integrity of interior bone structure. It is most commonly due to bacteria from the surface of the skin that invades a break in the skin and underlying tissue. In children, the rapidly growing areas of bone are most susceptible. In adults, diabetes is a common predisposing factor for osteomyelitis. Prosthetic joints are also at risk for infection.

How it happens

Typically, endogenous osteomyelitis occurs when organisms invade bone from recent trauma or in a weakened area, such as the site of local infection and travel through the bloodstream to the metaphysis, the section of a long bone that's continuous with the epiphysis plates, where the blood flows into sinusoids.

The most common pyogenic organism in osteomyelitis is *Staphylococcus aureus*, the common skin flora. Intraosseous or hematologic antibiotic treatment is essential. Diabetes is a major risk factor for osteomyelitis. In diabetes, there is impaired wound healing, diminished immunity, and decreased circulation, which increases the susceptibility of bone to infection, particularly in the lower extremities.

Stages of osteomyelitis

Initial infection

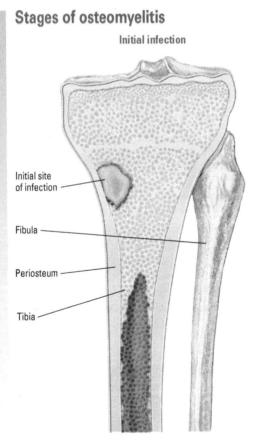

Initial site of infection

Fibula

Periosteum

Tibia

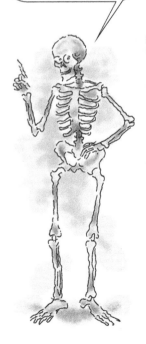

Although osteomyelitis typically remains localized, it can spread through the bone to the marrow, cortex, and periosteum.

What to look for

- Rapid onset with sudden pain in the affected bone
- Tenderness
- Warmth over region of infection
- Swelling
- Erythema
- Guarding of the affected region of the limb
- Restricted movement
- Chronic infection presenting intermittently for years, flaring after minor trauma or persisting as drainage of pus from an old pocket in a sinus tract
- Fever

age-old story

Age and osteomyelitis

Osteomyelitis is more common in children (especially boys) than in adults—usually as a complication of an acute localized infection. Typical sites in children are the lower end of the femur and the upper ends of the tibia, humerus, and radius. The most common sites in adults are the vertebrae and lower extremities generally after surgery or trauma.

Osteomyelitis is more common in children, especially boys. It is also common in patients with diabetic wound infection.

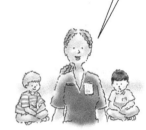

First stage

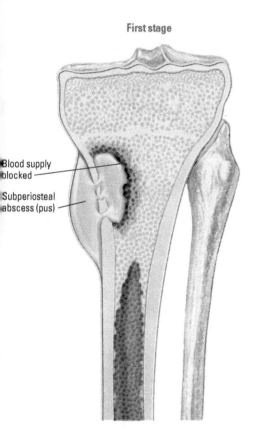

Blood supply blocked

Subperiosteal abscess (pus)

Second stage

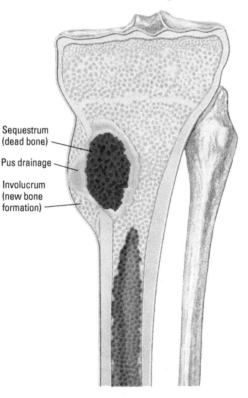

Sequestrum (dead bone)

Pus drainage

Involucrum (new bone formation)

Osteoporosis

Osteoporosis is a metabolic bone disorder in which the rate of bone resorption accelerates and the rate of bone formation decelerates. The result is decreased bone mass. Bones affected by this disease lose calcium and phosphate and become porous, brittle, and abnormally prone to fracture.

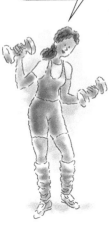

It's best to build those muscles and strengthen those bones to avoid osteoporosis.

How it happens

In normal bone, the rates of bone formation and resorption are constant; replacement follows resorption immediately, and the amount of bone replaced equals the amount of bone resorbed. Ca⁺⁺ is absorbed in the GI tract with facilitation by vitamin D. Ca⁺⁺ is then deposited in bone.

Osteoporosis develops when the remodeling cycle is interrupted, and new bone formation falls behind resorption. When bone is resorbed faster than it forms, the bone becomes less dense. Men have about 30% greater bone mass than women, which may explain why osteoporosis occurs most often in women and develops later in men.

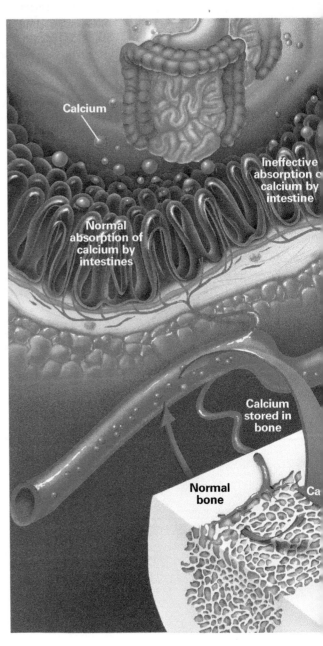

Calcium

Ineffective absorption of calcium by intestine

Normal absorption of calcium by intestines

Calcium stored in bone

Normal bone

Ca

Age and osteoporosis

Primary osteoporosis is often called *senile* or *postmenopausal* osteoporosis because it most commonly develops in postmenopausal women; estrogen supports normal bone metabolism.

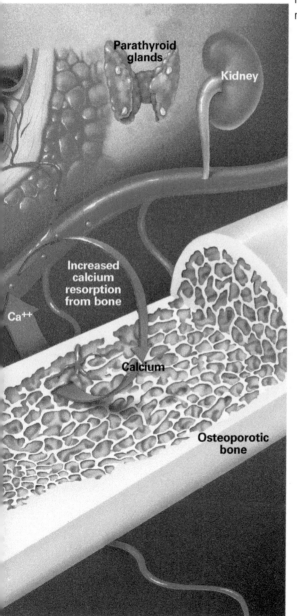

Parathyroid glands

Kidney

Increased calcium resorption from bone

Ca⁺⁺

Calcium

Osteoporotic bone

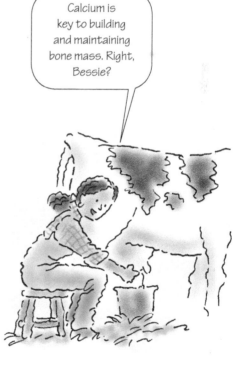

Calcium is key to building and maintaining bone mass. Right, Bessie?

What to look for

- Loss of height
- Spinal deformity (cervicothoracic kyphosis)
- Spontaneous vertebral compression fractures
- Fracture of wrist
- Fracture of head or neck of the femur (hip)
- Back pain

Bone formation and resorption

The organic portion of bone, called *osteoid,* acts as the matrix or framework for the mineral portion. Bone-forming cells, called *osteoblasts,* produce the osteoid matrix. The mineral portion, which consists of calcium and other minerals, hardens the osteoid matrix.

Large bone cells reshape mature bones by resorbing the mineral and organic components. However, in osteoporosis, osteoblasts continue to produce bone, but resorption by osteoclasts exceeds bone formation. There are 2 kinds of bone in the body: cortical (solid) bone and trabecular (mesh-like) bone. Trabecular bone undergoes effects of osteoporosis before solid bone and is most susceptible to fracture. Trabecular-type bone is in the wrist, hip, and vertebrae. Hip fracture is common in osteoporosis and can lead to fatal complications.

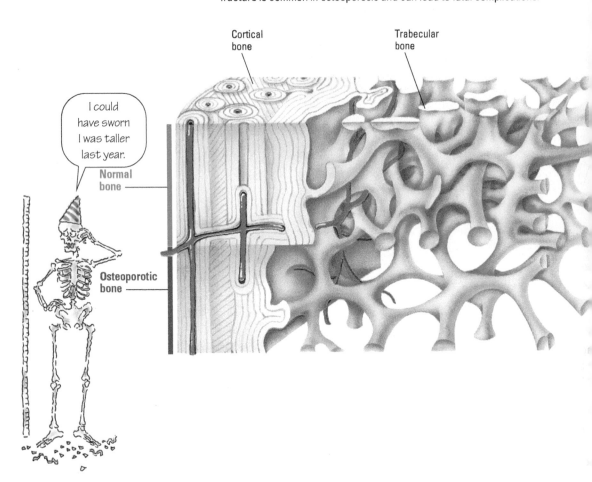

Cortical bone

Trabecular bone

I could have sworn I was taller last year.

Normal bone

Osteoporotic bone

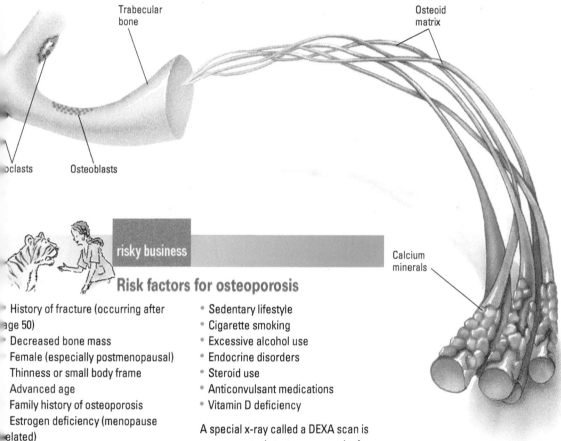

Trabecular bone

Osteoid matrix

oclasts

Osteoblasts

Calcium minerals

Risk factors for osteoporosis

- History of fracture (occurring after age 50)
- Decreased bone mass
- Female (especially postmenopausal)
- Thinness or small body frame
- Advanced age
- Family history of osteoporosis
- Estrogen deficiency (menopause related)
- Amenorrhea
- Anorexia nervosa or malnutrition
- Low lifetime calcium intake
- Low testosterone level (males)

- Sedentary lifestyle
- Cigarette smoking
- Excessive alcohol use
- Endocrine disorders
- Steroid use
- Anticonvulsant medications
- Vitamin D deficiency

A special x-ray called a DEXA scan is necessary to detect osteoporosis. A urine test for breakdown products of bone can also be used to detect osteoporosis.

Osteosarcoma

Osteosarcoma is a highly aggressive malignant bone tumor usually occurring during periods of bone growth. It most commonly occurs in the extremities of long bones near metaphyseal growth plates. Although it can occur in any bone, it tends to appear most frequently in bones that have the fastest bone growth, such as the lower femur or upper tibia or fibula. The humerus is the second most common site.

How it happens

Osteosarcomas are growths of abnormal cells in bones. These abnormal cells divide uncontrollably, and healthy tissue is replaced with unhealthy tissue. Osteosarcomas grow rapidly and move from the metaphysis of the bone to the periosteal surface.

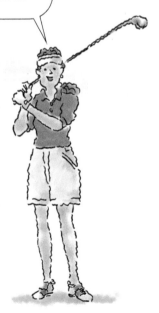

All *humerus* aside...the lower femur, upper tibia, and fibula (and humerus) are the *fore* sites most often affected by osteosarcoma.

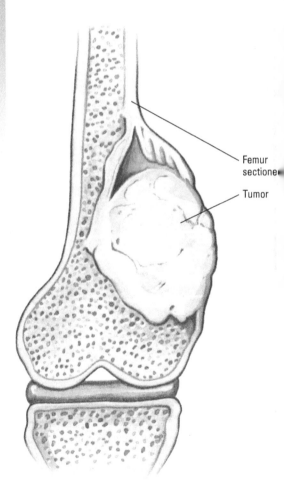

Femur sectioned

Tumor

Age and osteosarcoma

Osteosarcoma occurs commonly in adolescents, more often in males than females.

Osteosarcoma in the distal femur

In the distal femur, which is a very common site, osteosarcoma has extended through the cortex of the bone into the soft tissue and the bony epiphysis.

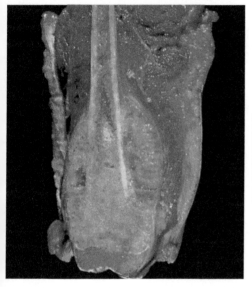

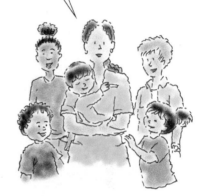

Osteosarcoma is the most common bone tumor in children.

What to look for

- Deep, localized pain
- Nighttime awakening with pain
- Swelling in the affected bone
- Sudden onset of pain
- Knee area is most common site

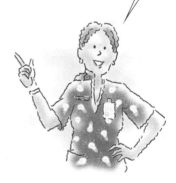

These are the five things to look for when checking for signs and symptoms of osteosarcomas.

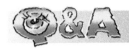

Able to label?

In this illustration, label the parts of the hand involved in carpal tunnel syndrome.

1. _____   2. _____   3. _____

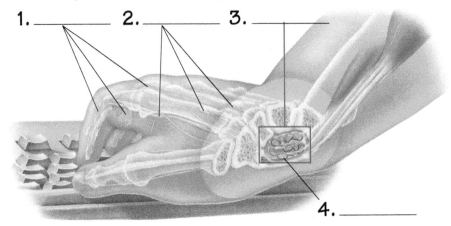

4. _____

My word!

Solve the word scrambles to identify parts of the musculoskeletal system. Then rearrange the circled letters to answer the question posed.

Question: What's the most common form of arthritis in adults?

1. gecailart _ _ _ ◯◯ _ _ _ ◯

2. tjnsoi _ ◯ _ _ ◯ _

3. regsnif _ ◯ _ _ _ ◯ _

4. nseke _ _ _ _ ◯

5. onbcsuladrh _ _ _ _ ◯ _ _ _ ◯◯ _

6. drchyoncoest _ _ ◯ _ _ _ _ _ ◯ _ ◯

Answer: _ _ _ _ _ _ _ _ _ _ _ _ _ _

Selected References

Barcenilla, A., March, L., Chen, J., & Sambrook, P. (2012). Carpal tunnel syndrome and its relationship to occupation: A meta-analysis. *Rheumatology, 51*(2), 250–261.

Beck-Broichsitter, B., Smeets, R., & Heiland, M. (2015). Current concepts in pathogenesis of acute and chronic osteo-myelitis. *Current Opinion in Infectious Diseases, 28*(3), 240–245.

Casazza, B. A. (2012). Diagnosis and treatment of acute low back pain. *American Family Physician, 85*(4), 343–350.

Duong, L. A., & Richardson, L. C. (2013). Descriptive epidemiology of malignant primary osteosarcoma using popula-tion-based registries, United States, 1999–2008. *Journal of Registry Management, 40*(2), 59–64.

Kanis, J., Odén, A., McCloskey, E., Johansson, H., Wahl, D., & Cooper, C. (2102). A systematic review of hip fracture incidence and probability of fracture worldwide. *Osteoporosis International, 23*(9), 2239–2256.

Kumar, V., Abbas, A., Fausto, N., & Aster, J. (2015). *Robbins & Cotran pathologic basis of disease* (9th ed.). New York, NY: Saunders.

LeBlanc, K. E., & Cestia, W. (2011). Carpal tunnel syndrome. *American Family Physician, 83*(8), 952–958.

Lotz, J., Haughton, V., Boden S., An, H. S., Kang, J. D., Masuda, K., ... Marinelli, N. L. (2012). New treatments and imaging strategies in degenerative disease of the intervertebral disks. *Radiology, 264*(1), 6–19.

Prieto-Alhambra, D., Judge, A., Javaid, M., Cooper, C., Diez-Perez, A., & Arden, M. (2014). Incidence and risk factors for clinically diagnosed knee, hip and hand osteoarthritis: Influences of age, gender and osteoarthritis affect-ing other joints. *Annals of the Rheumatic Diseases, 17*(9), 1659–1664.

Roth, E., Mirochna, M., & Harsha, D. (2012). Adolescent with knee pain. *American Family Physician, 86*(6), 569–570.

Sinusas, K. (2012). Osteoarthritis: Diagnosis and treatment. *American Family Physician, 85*(1), 49–56.

Hematologic disorders

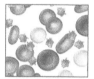

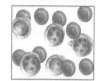
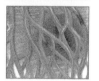
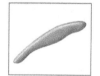

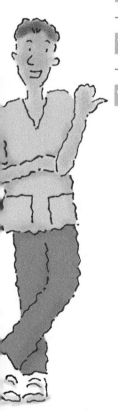

Anemia, folic acid deficiency

Hematologic

Folic acid deficiency anemia is a common, slowly progressive, megaloblastic anemia. In megaloblastic anemias, red blood cells are enlarged and do not carry oxygen very well.

How it happens

Folic acid is found in most body tissues, where it acts as a coenzyme in metabolic processes. It's essential for the formation and maturation of red blood cells (RBCs) and the synthesis of deoxyribonucleic acid. Although its body stores are relatively small (about 70 mg), this vitamin is plentiful in most well-balanced diets.

This deficiency inhibits cell growth, particularly RBCs, leading to production of few, deformed RBCs. These enlarged red cells characteristic of the megaloblastic anemias have a shortened life span—weeks rather than months. In pregnant women, folic acid deficiency causes defects in the central nervous system (CNS) of the fetus.

The lowdown on low folic acid

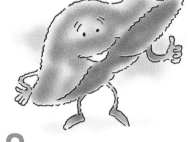

Get the point? I need my folic acid.

2 Depleted body stores in the liver

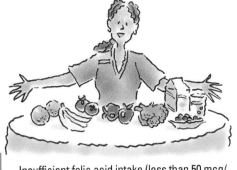

A well-balanced diet provides a healthy supply of folic acid.

1 Insufficient folic acid intake (less than 50 mcg/day) or malabsorption

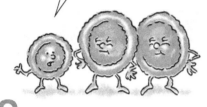

> Hey, you guys without folic acid are way bigger than me, but I can carry oxygen better!

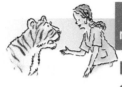

risky business

Risk factors for folic acid deficiency anemia

- Alcohol abuse
- Poor diet (lacking whole grains and green vegetables)
- Prolonged drug therapy (anticonvulsants, sulfonamides, and estrogens, including hormonal contraceptives)
- Pregnancy and breast-feeding
- Malignant or intestinal diseases that cause malabsorption

3 Inhibition of RBC growth

> Gasp! I don't want a shortened life span!

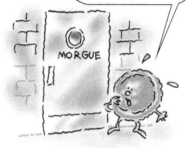

MORGUE

What to look for

- Anorexia
- Fainting
- Weakness
- Progressive fatigue
- Shortness of breath
- Palpitations
- Forgetfulness
- Glossitis (swollen tongue)
- Headache
- Irritability
- Nausea
- Pallor

> I may be bigger, but I don't carry oxygen as well as you normal-size RBCs!

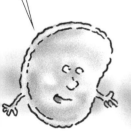

4 Production of few, deformed, enlarged RBCs called megaloblasts.

> Take A SWING at some signs and symptoms of folic acid deficiency.

5 RBCs deficient in folic acid have short life span and cannot carry oxygen well.

memory board

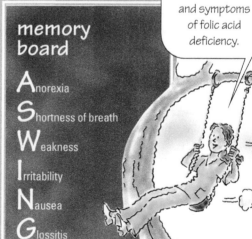

Anorexia
Shortness of breath
Weakness
Irritability
Nausea
Glossitis

Anemia, iron deficiency

Iron deficiency anemia causes lack of optimal hemoglobin (Hgb) production. Lack of sufficient Hgb leads to decreased oxygen carriage by red blood cells. A common disease worldwide, iron deficiency anemia affects 10% to 30% of the adult population of the United States. The prognosis after replacement therapy is favorable.

How it happens

Iron deficiency anemia occurs when the supply of iron is too low for optimal Hgb formation. The low iron supply results in smaller (microcytic) cells that contain less color (hypochromic) when they're stained for visualization under a microscope. The decreased Hgb creates RBCs that cannot carry the optimal amount of oxygen needed for the tissues.

Peripheral blood smear in iron deficiency anemia

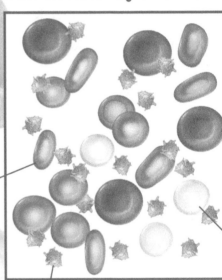

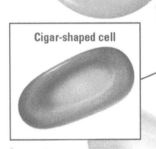
Cigar-shaped cell

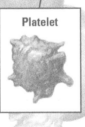
Platelet

I knew I should have taken my iron today.

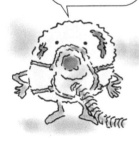

Age and iron deficiency anemia

Iron deficiency anemia is most common in premenopausal women, infants (particularly premature or low-birth-weight infants), children, adolescents (especially girls), and older adults who eat poorly.

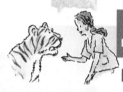

risky business

Risk factors for iron deficiency anemia

Insufficient intake of iron
- Vegetarian diet
- Macrobiotic diet
- Low intake of meat, fish, poultry, or iron-fortified foods (including conditions resulting in malabsorption)
- Low intake of foods rich in ascorbic acid (vitamin C enhances absorption of iron)
- Frequent dieting or restricted eating
- Chronic or significant weight loss
- Weaning children from breast milk to cow's milk (cow's milk is a poor iron source)

Excessive loss of iron
- Heavy or lengthy menstrual periods
- Rapid growth
- Pregnancy (recent or current)
- Inflammatory bowel disease
- Colon cancer (causes gastrointestinal bleeding)
- Chronic use of aspirin or nonsteroidal anti-inflammatory drugs (NSAIDs), such as ibuprofen, that can cause gastrointestinal bleeding
- Corticosteroid use
- Participation in endurance sports (long-distance running, swimming, cycling)

Normal RBC

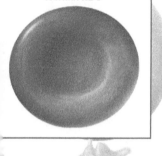

Microcytic, hypochromic RBC

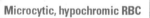

What to look for

- Pallor
- Exertional dyspnea
- Fatigue
- Weakness
- Tachycardia, which causes palpitations
- Coarsely ridged, spoon-shaped (koilonychia), brittle, thin nails
- Sore, red, burning tongue
- Sore, dry skin in the corners of the mouth
- Hair loss
- PICA (craving of nonfood items, e.g., ice, chalk)

Anemia, pernicious

Pernicious anemia, the most common type of megaloblastic anemia, is caused by malabsorption of vitamin B_{12}. It's characterized by a lack of intrinsic factor, which is needed to absorb vitamin B_{12} in the intestine.

Lack of vitamin B_{12} causes neurologic deficits such as gait and balance disturbances, numbness and tingling in the lower extremities, and cognitive impairment (dementia).

How it happens

Pernicious anemia is characterized by decreased production of intrinsic factor, which is normally secreted by the parietal cells of the gastric mucosa and is essential for vitamin B_{12} absorption in the ileum. The resulting vitamin B_{12} deficiency inhibits cell growth, particularly of RBCs, leading to production of few, enlarged RBCs with poor oxygen-carrying capacity. It also causes neurologic damage by impairing myelin formation.

Peripheral blood smear in pernicious anemia

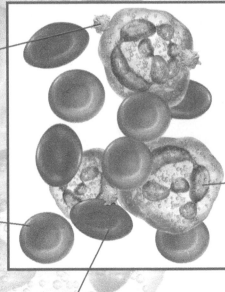

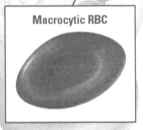

Platelet

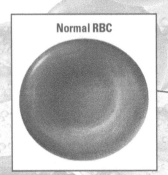

Normal RBC

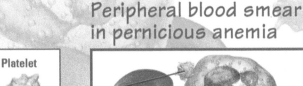

Macrocytic RBC

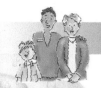

Age and pernicious anemia

The onset of pernicious anemia typically occurs in older adults. Elderly patients commonly have a dietary deficiency of vitamin B_{12} in addition to poor absorption.

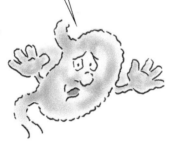

I'd feel much better with a little help from my friend intrinsic factor.

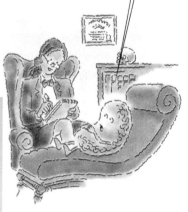

It all started when my myelin broke down.

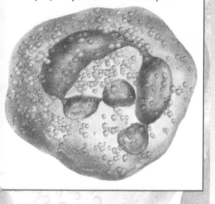

Hypersegmented polymorphonuclear neutrophil

What to look for

White blood cells
Nucleus of WBCs becomes hypersegmented

Neurologic
* Neuritis and weakness in the extremities
* Peripheral numbness and paresthesia
* Disturbed position sense
* Lack of coordination, ataxia, and impaired fine finger movement
* Positive Babinski and Romberg signs
* Light-headedness
* Altered vision (diplopia, blurred vision), taste, smell, and hearing (tinnitus), and optic muscle atrophy
* Irritability, poor memory, headache, depression, and delirium

Cardiovascular
* Low hemoglobin level
* Palpitations
* Dyspnea
* Tachycardia

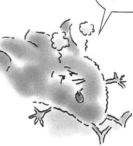

Hey! I shouldn't be doing all the work. Where are those RBCs?

Disseminated intravascular coagulation

> Early detection is crucial! Prognosis depends on it as well as the severity of the hemorrhage and the treatment of the underlying disease.

Disseminated intravascular coagulation (DIC), also called *consumption coagulopathy*, is a complication of a disease or condition that accelerates clotting throughout the body. This accelerated clotting causes small blood vessel occlusion, organ necrosis, depletion of circulating clotting factors and platelets, activation of the fibrinolytic system, and consequent severe hemorrhage. In DIC, the coagulation system becomes dysfunctional; there are episodes of clotting and bleeding.

Clotting in the microcirculation (small blood vessels) usually affects the kidneys and extremities but may occur in the brain, lungs, pituitary and adrenal glands, and GI mucosa. DIC is generally an acute condition but may be chronic in cancer patients.

How it happens

It isn't clear how or why certain disorders lead to DIC. In many patients, the triggering mechanisms may be the entrance of foreign protein into the circulation and vascular endothelial injury. It usually occurs in critically ill patients.

Regardless of how DIC begins, the typical accelerated clotting results in generalized activation of prothrombin and a consequent excess of thrombin.

Tissue damage in DIC

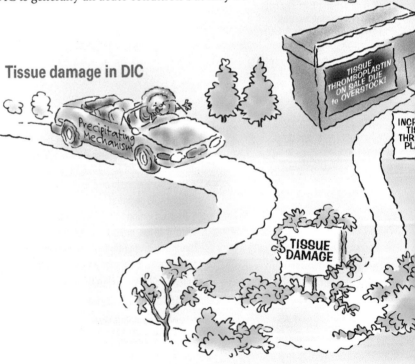

TISSUE THROMBOPLASTIN ON SALE DUE to OVERSTOCK!

Precipitating Mechanism

TISSUE DAMAGE

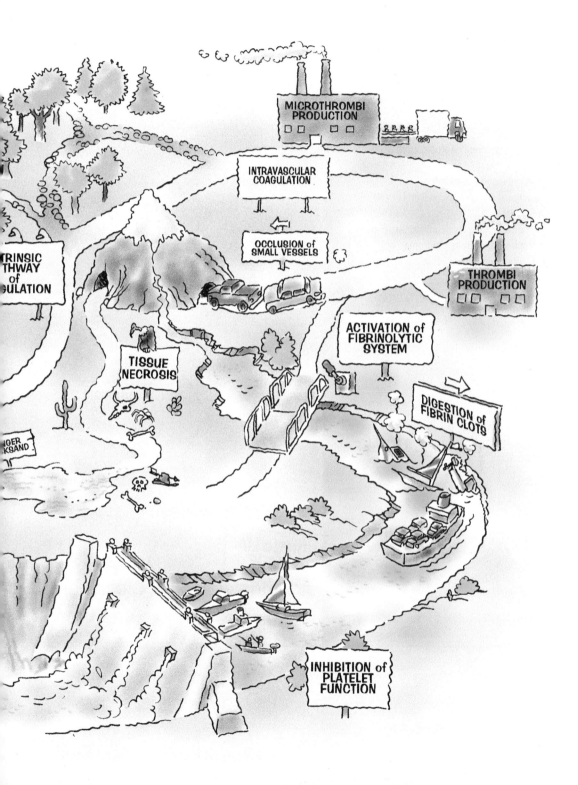

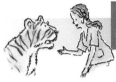

Risk factors for DIC

- Infection
- Obstetric complications
- Neoplastic disease
- Disorders that produce necrosis, such as extensive burns and trauma
- Shock
- Incompatible blood transfusions
- Drug reactions
- Cardiac arrest
- Surgery necessitating cardiopulmonary bypass
- Acute respiratory distress syndrome
- Diabetic ketoacidosis
- Pulmonary embolism
- Severe liver disease
- Severe head injury

Endothelial damage in DIC

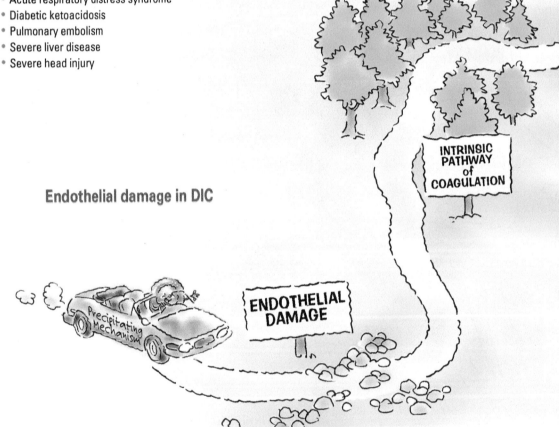

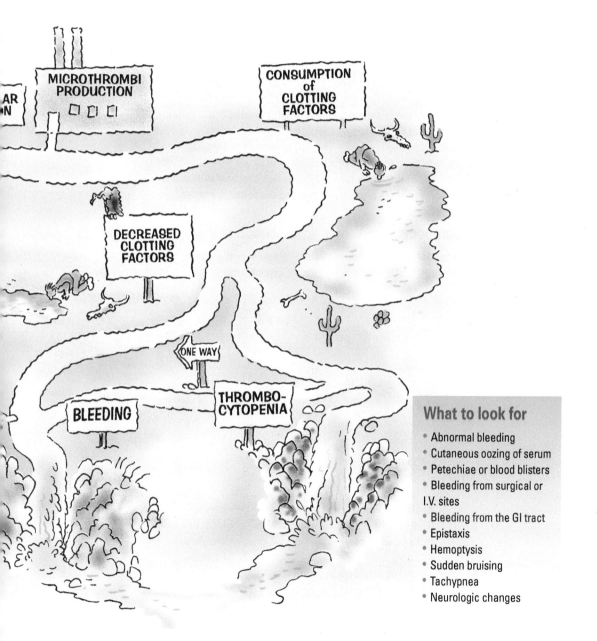

What to look for

- Abnormal bleeding
- Cutaneous oozing of serum
- Petechiae or blood blisters
- Bleeding from surgical or I.V. sites
- Bleeding from the GI tract
- Epistaxis
- Hemoptysis
- Sudden bruising
- Tachypnea
- Neurologic changes

Leukemia

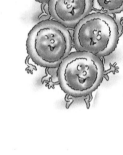

> When leukemic cells crowd up, it tends to mean trouble. We get shoved out, and pancytopenia results.

Leukemia refers to a group of malignant disorders characterized by abnormal proliferation of white blood cells in the bone marrow, leading to the suppression of normal blood cells. It can be classified as *acute* or *chronic*, with subclassifications of *lymphocytic* or *myelogenous*.

How it happens

In leukemia, hematopoietic cells (immature blood cells) undergo an abnormal transformation, giving rise to leukemic cells. Leukemic cells rapidly multiply and accumulate, crowding out other types of cells. Crowding prevents production of normal red and white blood cells and platelets, leading to pancytopenia (reduced number of all cellular elements of the blood). Lack of normal numbers of RBCs causes anemia, lack of normal WBCs causes infections, and lack of platelets causes bruising and bleeding due to inability to clot.

Acute lymphocytic leukemia

Abnormal growth of lymphocytic precursors (lymphoblasts)

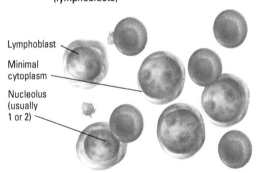

Lymphoblast

Minimal cytoplasm

Nucleolus (usually 1 or 2)

Acute myelogenous leukemia

Rapid accumulation of myeloid precursors (myeloblasts)

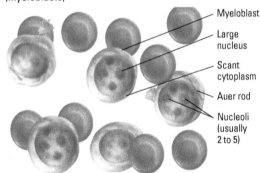

Myeloblast

Large nucleus

Scant cytoplasm

Auer rod

Nucleoli (usually 2 to 5)

What to look for

Acute (lymphocytic and myeloid)
Related to suppression of all blood cells in the bone marrow
- Anemia
- Bleeding (nosebleeds, gums bleeding)
- Easy bruising
- Fever

- Infection
- Night sweats
- Weight loss
- Paleness
- Lethargy
- Malaise

Age and leukemia

Acute lymphocytic leukemia accounts for 80% of childhood cases of leukemia. Treatment leads to remission in 81% of children, who survive an average of 5 years, and in 65% of adults, who survive an average of 2 years. Children ages 2 to 8 who receive intensive therapy have the best survival rate.

> Smoking, along with exposure to certain chemicals, drugs, or ionizing radiation, can cause leukemia.

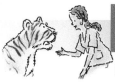

Risk factors for leukemia

- Cigarette smoking
- Exposure to certain chemicals (such as benzene, which is present in cigarette smoke and gasoline)
- Exposure to large doses of ionizing radiation or drugs that depress the bone marrow (such as chemotherapy)

Chronic lymphocytic leukemia

Uncontrollable spread of small, abnormal lymphocytes in lymphoid tissue, blood, and bone marrow

Chronic myelogenous leukemia

Abnormal overgrowth of granulocytic precursors (myeloblasts, promyelocytes, metamyelocytes, and myelocytes) in bone marrow, blood, and body tissue

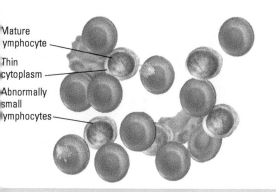

Mature lymphocyte

Thin cytoplasm

Abnormally small lymphocytes

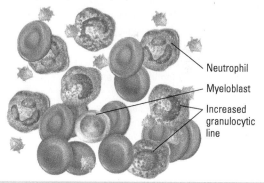

Neutrophil

Myeloblast

Increased granulocytic line

Chronic lymphocytic

Early
- Fatigue
- Malaise
- Fever
- Nodular enlargement

Late
- Bone tenderness
- Liver or spleen enlargement
- Severe fatigue
- Weight loss

Chronic myelogenous
- Anemia
- Thrombocytopenia
- Ankle edema
- Anorexia, weight loss
- Hepatosplenomegaly
- Prolonged infection
- Low-grade fever
- Renal calculi or gouty arthritis
- Sternal and rib tenderness
- Increased sweating

Sickle cell disease

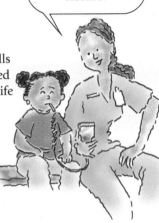

Race has a lot to do with susceptibility to sickle cell disease.

Sickle cell disease is a congenital hemolytic anemia resulting from defective hemoglobin molecules. It is due to a genetic defect that causes red blood cells to change into a sickle shape. In the past, patients with sickle cell disease died in their early 20s, and few lived to middle age. Today, however, the average life expectancy is age 45, with 40% to 50% of patients living into their 50s.

Sickle cell disease occurs primarily in persons of African and Mediterranean descent, but it also affects other populations, such as those indigenous to Puerto Rico, Turkey, India, and the Middle East. About 1 in 12 blacks carries the abnormal gene, and 1 in every 400 to 600 black children has sickle cell disease.

How it happens

Sickle cell disease results from the substitution of the amino acid valine for glutamic acid in the hemoglobin S gene, which is an abnormality found in the RBCs of patients with sickle cell disease and which becomes insoluble during hypoxia. As a result, these blood cells become rigid, rough, and elongated, forming a sickle (crescent) shape, which causes hemolysis (disintegration of the cell and release of hemoglobin). The altered cells also pile up in the capillaries and smaller blood vessels, making the blood more viscous. Normal circulation is impaired, causing pain, tissue ischemia, and organ infarctions.

Each patient with sickle cell disease has a different hypoxic threshold and different factors that trigger a sickle cell crisis, in which the sickled blood cells block small blood vessels. Illness, exposure to cold, stress, acidosis, or dehydration precipitates a crisis in most patients. The blood vessel blockages then cause anoxic changes that lead to further sickling and obstruction.

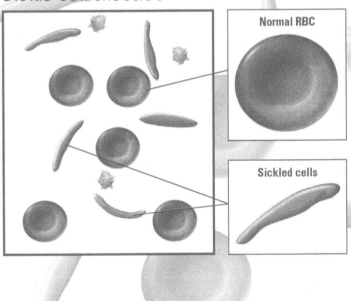

Blood smear in sickle cell disease

Normal RBC

Sickled cells

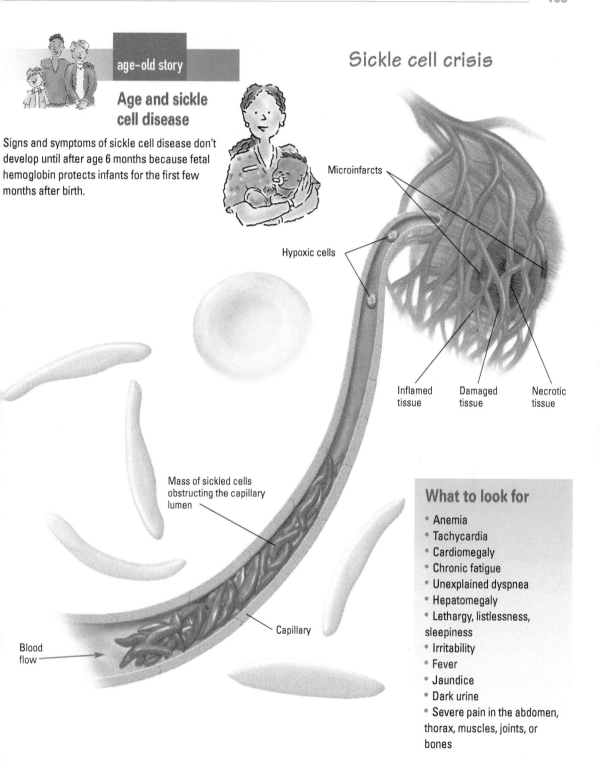

Age and sickle cell disease

Signs and symptoms of sickle cell disease don't develop until after age 6 months because fetal hemoglobin protects infants for the first few months after birth.

Sickle cell crisis

Microinfarcts

Hypoxic cells

Inflamed tissue

Damaged tissue

Necrotic tissue

Mass of sickled cells obstructing the capillary lumen

Capillary

Blood flow

What to look for

- Anemia
- Tachycardia
- Cardiomegaly
- Chronic fatigue
- Unexplained dyspnea
- Hepatomegaly
- Lethargy, listlessness, sleepiness
- Irritability
- Fever
- Jaundice
- Dark urine
- Severe pain in the abdomen, thorax, muscles, joints, or bones

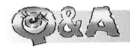

Show and tell

Identify the four types of leukemia shown in these illustrations and differentiate among them.

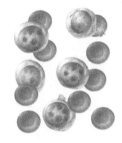 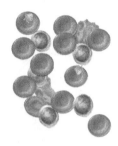 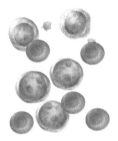 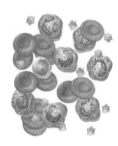

1. _____   2. _____   3. _____   4. _____

_____   _____   _____   _____

_____   _____   _____   _____

_____   _____   _____   _____

Matchmaker

Match the definitions in column 1 with the disorder terms in column 2.

1. Disorder of oxygen transport in which hemoglobin synthesis is deficient

2. Common, slowly progressive, megaloblastic anemia _____

3. Congenital hemolytic anemia resulting from defective hemoglobin molecules _____

4. Complication of a disease or condition that accelerates clotting _____

5. Most common type of megaloblastic anemia; caused by malabsorption of vitamin B_{12} _____

6. Group of malignant disorders characterized by abnormal proliferation and maturation of lymphocytes and nonlymphocytic cells _____

A. Folic acid deficiency anemia

B. Iron deficiency anemia

C. Pernicious anemia

D. DIC

E. Leukemia

F. Sickle cell disease

Answers: Show and tell: 1. acute myelogenous, rapid accumulation of myeloblasts; 2. chronic lymphocytic, uncontrollable spread of small, abnormal lymphocytes; 3. acute lymphocytic, abnormal growth of lymphoblasts; 4. chronic myeloid, abnormal overgrowth of granulocyte precursors. Matchmaker 1. B, 2. A, 3. F, 4. E, 5. C, 6. E.

Selected References

Bross, M. H., Soch, K., & Smith-Knuppel, T. (2010). Anemia in older persons. *American Family Physician, 82*(5), 480–487.

Centers for Disease Control and Prevention. (2011, September 16). Sickle cell disease data and statistics. Retrieved from: http://www.cdc.gov/ncbddd/sicklecell/data.html on May 3, 2015.

Davis, A. S., Viera, A. J., & Mead, M. D. (2014). Leukemia: An overview for primary care. *American Family Physician, 89*(9), 731–738.

Langan, R. C., & Zawistoski, K. J. (2011). Update on vitamin B12 deficiency. *American Family Physician, 83*(12), 1425–1430.

National Cancer Institute. (2015, June 8). Acute adult lymphoblastic leukemia. Retrieved from: http://www. cancer.gov/types/leukemia/patient/adult-all-treatment-pdq#section/_1 on May 3, 2015.

Rees, D. C., Williams, T. N., & Gladwin, M. T. (2010). Sickle-cell disease. *Lancet, 376*(9757), 2018–2031.

Short, M. W., & Domagalski, J. E. (2013). Iron deficiency anemia: Evaluation and management. *American Family Physician, 87*(2), 98–104.

United States Library of Medicine. (2013, September 13). Folate deficiency. Retrieved from: http://www.nlm.nih.gov/medlineplus/ency/article/000354.htm on May 2, 2015.

Immune disorders

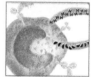
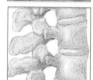
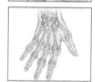
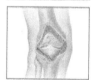
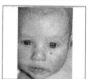
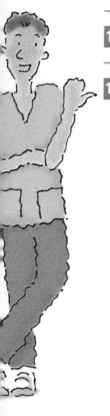

Acquired immunodeficiency syndrome

Immune

Acquired immunodeficiency syndrome (AIDS) is thought to be caused by human immunodeficiency virus (HIV) infection. HIV is characterized by gradual destruction of CD4 cells (also called T helper cells) over time. AIDS is diagnosed after the CD4 (also called T helper cell) count has declined below 200 cells/mm³. HIV targets the CD4+ cells that play a central role in the two major types of immunity: humoral immunity and cell-mediated immunity.

How immunity works: we have two types of immunity that work differently to defend the body

Humoral immunity
When foreign substances (antigens) invade the body, B lymphocytes secrete antibodies that attack the antigen; this is called an *antibody-mediated response, also called B-cell immunity.*

Antibody-mediated immunity requires CD4 cells to accomplish destruction of the antigen; therefore, when HIV attacks CD4 cells, antibody-mediated (B-cell) immunity is inactivated.

Cell-mediated immunity
When foreign substances (antigen) invade the body, CD4 and CD8 T lymphocytes (also called T helper cells and cytotoxic T cells) directly attack the antigen; this is *also called T-cell immunity.*

Cell-mediated immunity requires CD4 cells to accomplish destruction of the antigen; therefore, when HIV attacks CD4 cells, cell-mediated immunity is inactivated.

How HIV deactivates the two major types of immunity
By destroying the CD4 cell, HIV causes deactivation of both humoral and cell-mediated immunity, which makes the patient susceptible to opportunistic infections, cancers, and other abnormalities that characterize AIDS. A CD4 cell is a T helper cell that takes part in the two types of immune reactions.

How it happens

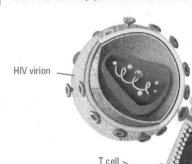

HIV virion

T cell

HIV life cycle

1 HIV binds to the T helper cell (also called CD4 cell).

2 Viral ribonucleic acid (RNA) is released into the host cell.

3 The viral RNA is converted into viral deoxyribonucleic acid (DNA) through an enzyme called reverse transcriptase. Reverse transcriptase reads the sequence of viral RNA nucleic acids that have entered the host cell and transcribes the sequence into a complementary DNA sequence.

4 Viral DNA enters the T helper cell's nucleus and integrates itself into the T cell genome.

5 The T helper cell begins to make copies of the HIV components.

6 Protease (an enzyme) helps create new virus particles.

7 The new HIV virion (virus particle) is released from the T helper cell.

8 The T helper cell dies.

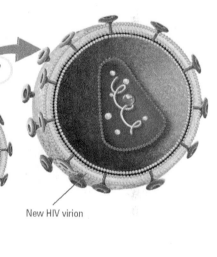

New HIV virion

Viral RNA

Reverse transcriptase

Viral DNA

Viral RNA

HIV proteins

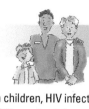

age-old story

HIV and children

In children, HIV infection has a mean incubation time of 17 months. Infants can acquire HIV infection in utero, during the birth process, or through breast-feeding.

Children affected by HIV have a high incidence of bacterial infections, such as otitis media, sepsis, chronic salivary gland enlargement, and opportunistic infections. Opportunistic infections include *Mycobacterium avium-intracellulare* infection and types of pneumonias, including lymphoid interstitial pneumonia and *Pneumocystis jiroveci* pneumonia (previously called *Pneumocystis carinii*).

Stages of HIV infection

1. Acute stage

The acute or primary stage of HIV occurs about 1 to 2 weeks after initial infection. During this stage, the virus undergoes massive replication. HIV antibody testing may be negative because it can take up to 2 months for the immune system to make enough antibodies for the test to detect them. The patient may be asymptomatic or have flulike symptoms.

2. Asymptomatic HIV

During the asymptomatic stage, chronic signs and symptoms may not be present. CD4 cell (also called T helper cell) count is used to monitor progression of the disease. With the patient's own immune response and drug therapy, this stage can last for 10 to 12 years or longer.

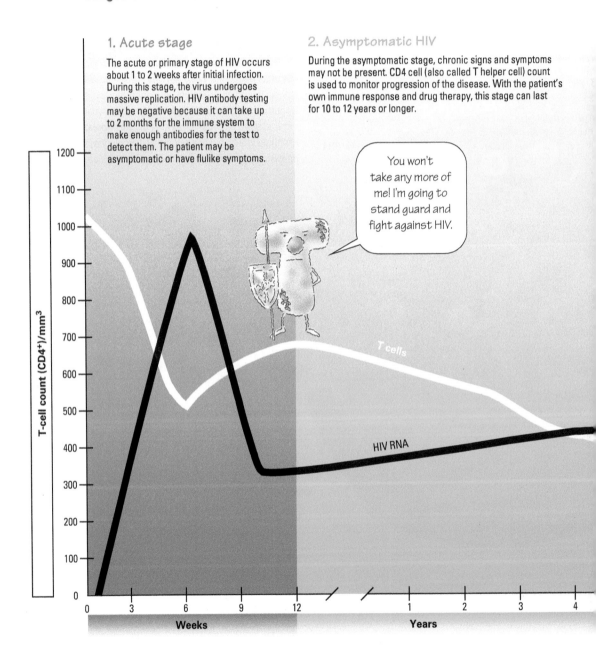

You won't take any more of me! I'm going to stand guard and fight against HIV.

T cells

HIV RNA

T-cell count (CD4⁺)/mm³

1200
1100
1000
900
800
700
600
500
400
300
200
100
0

0   3   6   9   12   1   2   3   4

Weeks   **Years**

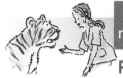

Risk factors for HIV infection

- Sexual contact with HIV-infected persons (with or without the use of condoms)
- Exposure to contaminated blood or contaminated needles or syringes
- Received a blood transfusion in the United States before 1986, or received a blood transfusion outside of the United States.
- Transplacental transmission to fetus
- Mother who has HIV infection can transfer HIV to infant during breast-feeding
- Transplant from an HIV+ donor

Symptomatic HIV

symptomatic stage has two phases:
and late. When the CD4 cell count in
d falls below 200 cells/mm³, it's the late
se or AIDS (acquired immunodeficiency
rome). This stage of HIV infection
fined mainly by the emergence of
rtunistic infections and cancers
hich the immune system normally
s maintain resistance.

---

4. Advanced HIV

A CD4 cell count of 50 cells/mm³ or less represents advanced HIV/AIDS. With the onset of this phase, a person's immune system is severely damaged and has difficulty fighting diseases and some cancers; this is when patients are at the highest risk for opportunistic infections and malignancies.

HIV RNA copies per ml plasma

10^7

10^6

10^5

10^4

10^3

10^2

7 8 9 10 11

What to look for

- High fever
- Sore throat
- Persistent or frequent oral infections (thrush, oral yeast infection)
- Difficulty or pain with swallowing (thrush, esophageal yeast infection)
- Loss of appetite
- Cough and shortness of breath
- Swollen lymph nodes in the neck, armpits, and groin
- Kaposi sarcoma (blood vessel tumors that appear as purple blotches on skin)
- Severe weight loss
- Chronic diarrhea
- Lack of energy and muscle weakness
- Chronic vaginal yeast infections
- Chronic pneumonia
- Tuberculosis
- Other sexually transmitted diseases

Allergic rhinitis

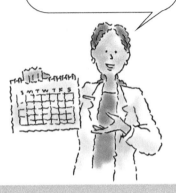

Allergic rhinitis can occur seasonally, such as with hay fever, or year-round, such as allergy to dust, animal dander, mold, or environmental allergens.

Allergic rhinitis is a reaction to airborne (inhaled) allergens. It's the most common allergic reaction, affecting more than 20 million Americans. Rhinitis (inflammation of the nasal mucous membrane) and conjunctivitis (inflammation of the conjunctiva) may occur seasonally or year-round.

How it happens

Allergic rhinitis may occur from primary exposure or reexposure.

Primary exposure

During primary exposure to an allergen, T cells recognize the foreign allergens and release chemicals that instruct B cells to produce specific antibodies called immuno-globulin E (IgE). IgE antibodies attach themselves to mast cells in the respiratory mucosa and to eosinophils and basophils in the peripheral blood. Stimulated mast cells, eosino-phils, and basophils secrete large amounts of histamine, serotonin, and leukotrienes, which cause a body-wide allergic reaction. Mast cells with attached IgE can remain in the body for years, ready to react when they next encounter the same allergen.

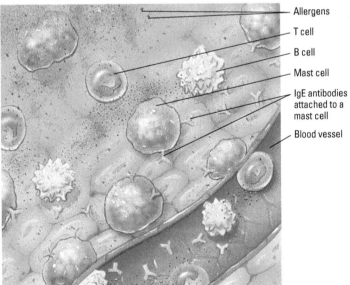

- Allergens
- T cell
- B cell
- Mast cell
- IgE antibodies attached to a mast cell
- Blood vessel

Age and allergic rhinitis

Allergic rhinitis is most prevalent in young children, adolescents, and young adults.

What to look for

Seasonal

- Paroxysmal sneezing; profuse, watery rhinorrhea (nasal mucus discharge); nasal obstruction or congestion; and itchy nose and eyes
- Pale, cyanotic, edematous nasal mucosa
- Red, edematous eyelids and conjunctiva
- Excessive lacrimation
- Headache or sinus pain
- Itching in the throat and malaise
- Dark circles under the eyes (allergic shiners)
- Bronchoconstriction (cough)

Perennial

- Postnasal drip, cough, fatigue
- Chronic nasal obstruction
- Allergic shiners

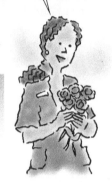

Roses are red, violets are blue, if I put these near me, I say "Achoo."

Reexposure

The second time the allergen enters the body, it comes into direct contact with the IgE antibodies attached to the mast cells. This contact stimulates the mast cells to release chemicals (such as histamine), which initiate a response that causes tightening of the smooth muscles in the airways, dilation of small blood vessels, increased mucus secretion in the nasal cavity and airways, and itching.

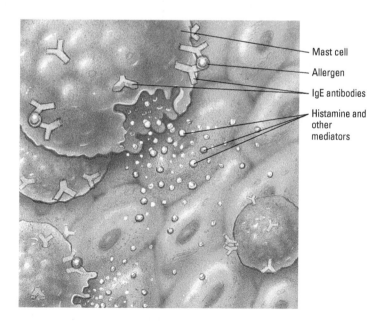

Mast cell

Allergen

IgE antibodies

Histamine and other mediators

Anaphylaxis

> With prompt treatment, the prognosis for anaphylaxis is good. But a severe reaction may lead to systemic shock and sometimes death.

Anaphylaxis is an acute, potentially life-threatening type I (immediate) hypersensitivity reaction marked by the sudden onset of rapidly progressive urticaria (hives) and respiratory distress. With prompt recognition and treatment, the prognosis is good. However, a severe reaction may precipitate vascular collapse, leading to severe hypotension, systemic shock, and, sometimes, death. The reaction typically occurs within minutes but can occur up to 1 hour after exposure to the antigen.

How it happens

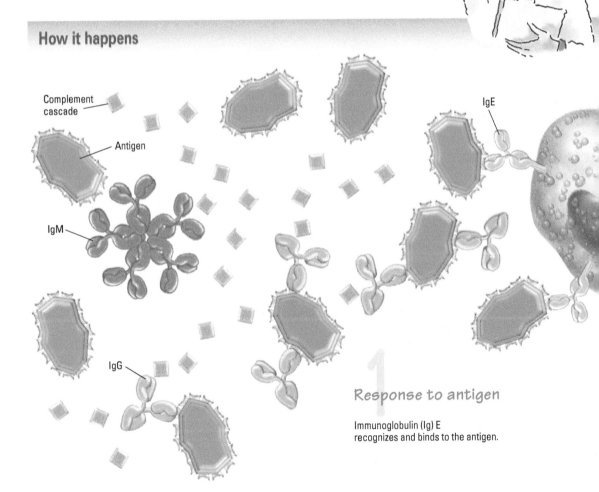

Complement cascade

Antigen

IgM

IgG

IgE

Response to antigen

Immunoglobulin (Ig) E recognizes and binds to the antigen.

Age and anaphylaxis

Children are more likely to experience food-related anaphylaxis. Adults are more likely to experience anaphylaxis related to antibiotics, radiocontrast media, anesthetic agents, and insect stings.

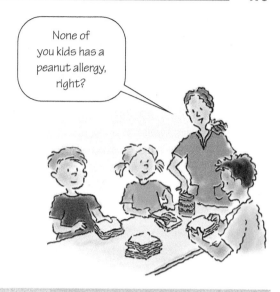

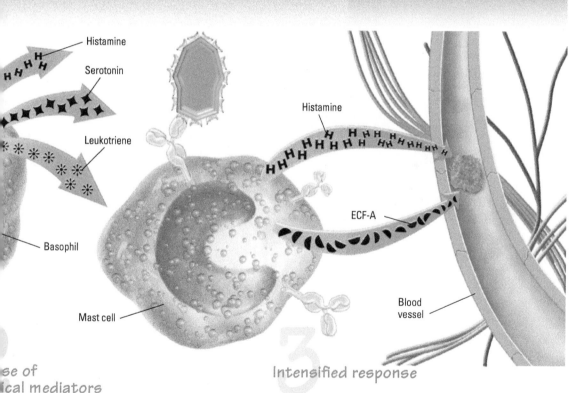

se of
ical mediators

IgE lands eosinophils and basophils and promotes se of mediators: histamine, serotonin, and leukotrienes.

Intensified response

Mast cells are stimulated by IgE and release more histamine and other inflammatory mediators.

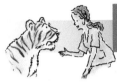

risky business

Risk factors for anaphylaxis

- History of allergies, eczema, or asthma
- Prior allergic reactions
- Prior anaphylactic reactions

What to look for

Initial
- Feeling of impending doom or fright
- Sweating
- Throat tightness
- Shortness of breath
- Urticaria (itchy hives)
- Facial swelling (angioedema)

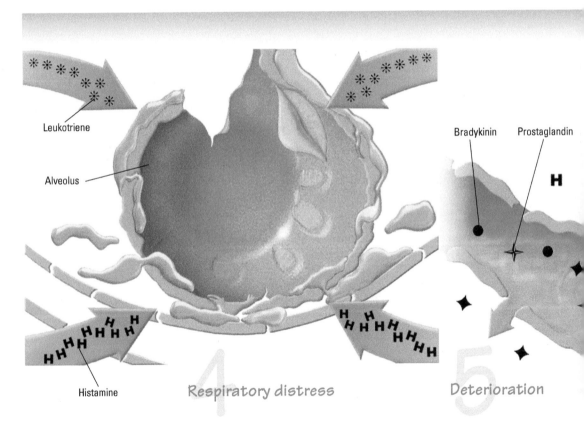

Leukotriene

Alveolus

Histamine

Bradykinin   Prostaglandin

H

Respiratory distress

In the lungs, histamine causes bronchial constriction, endothelial cell destruction, and fluid to leak into alveoli.

Deterioration

Meanwhile, mediators increase v permeability, causing fluid to leak vessels. The face and tongue ca severely swollen. Blood vessels throughout the body causing severely low BP and shock.

Systemic

- Hypotension, shock, and, sometimes, cardiac arrhythmias
- Nasal mucosal edema; profuse, watery rhinorrhea; itching; nasal congestion; and sudden sneezing attacks
- Edema of the upper respiratory tract, resulting in pharyngeal and laryngeal obstruction
- Hoarseness, stridor, wheezing, and accessory muscle use
- Tongue and facial swelling (called angioedema)

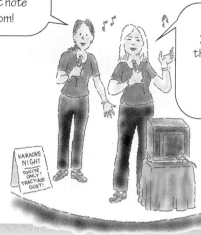

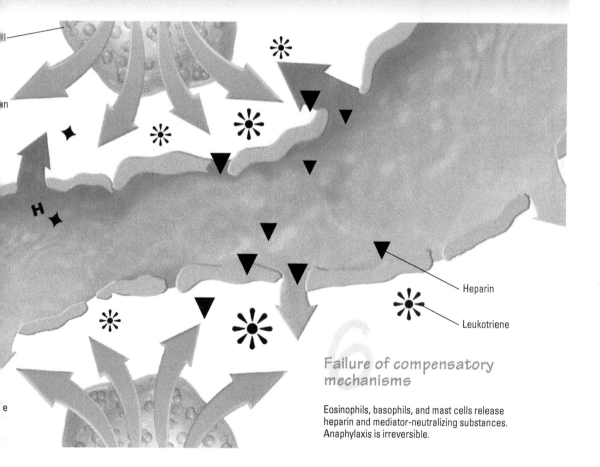

Failure of compensatory mechanisms

Eosinophils, basophils, and mast cells release heparin and mediator-neutralizing substances. Anaphylaxis is irreversible.

Heparin

Leukotriene

Ankylosing spondylitis

Ankylosing spondylitis is an autoimmune, chronic, progressive inflammatory bone disease that primarily affects the sacroiliac, apophyseal, and costovertebral joints along with the adjacent soft tissue. The disease usually begins in the sacroiliac joints and gradually progresses to the lumbar, thoracic, and cervical regions of the spine. Deterioration of the bone and cartilage can lead to formation of fibrous tissue and eventual fusion of the spine or the peripheral joints.

Spinal fusion in ankylosing spondylitis

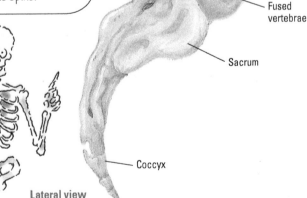

L1 — Normal vertebrae

L2 — Intervertebral disk

L3

L4

L5 — Fused vertebrae

Sacrum

Coccyx

Lateral view

How it happens

Fibrous tissue of the joint capsule is infiltrated by inflammatory cells that erode the bone and fibrocartilage. Repair of the cartilaginous structures begins with the proliferation of fibroblasts, which synthesize and secrete collagen. The collagen forms fibrous scar tissue that eventually undergoes calcification and ossification, causing the joint to fuse or lose flexibility. The result is ultimate destruction of these joints with fusion of the spine. The vertebrae have a squared appearance, sometimes referred to as "bamboo spine"; bones fuse one vertebral body to the next across the intervertebral disks.

Ankylosing spondylitis usually begins in the sacroiliac joints and progresses to the lumbar, thoracic, and cervical regions of the spine.

A closer look

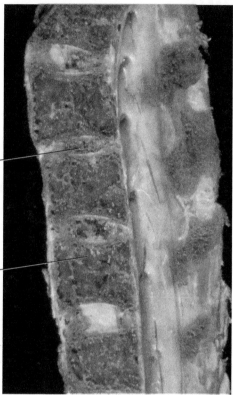

Intervertebral
disk replaced
by marrow

Osteoporosis
from disease

What to look for

• Intermittent lower back pain (more severe in the morning or after inactivity and relieved by exercise)
• Mild fatigue, fever, anorexia, weight loss
• Pain in the shoulders, hips, knees, and ankles
• Pain over the symphysis pubis
• Stiffness or limited motion of the lumbar spine
• Warmth, swelling, or tenderness of the affected joints

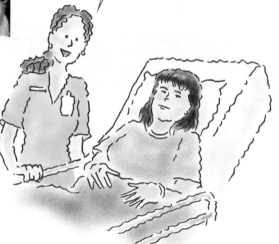

Pain in the lower back, shoulders, hips, knees, and ankles? Ankylosing spondylitis might be the culprit!

Atopic dermatitis

Atopic dermatitis, also referred to as *eczema*, is a chronic skin disorder characterized by superficial skin inflammation and intense pruritus (itching). Although this disorder may appear at any age, it typically begins during infancy or early childhood. It may then subside spontaneously, followed by exacerbations in late childhood, adolescence, or early adulthood.

Age and atopic dermatitis

About 10% of childhood cases of atopic dermatitis are caused by allergy to certain foods, especially eggs, milk, peanuts, and wheat.

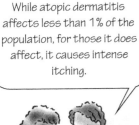

While atopic dermatitis affects less than 1% of the population, for those it does affect, it causes intense itching.

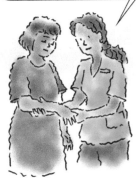

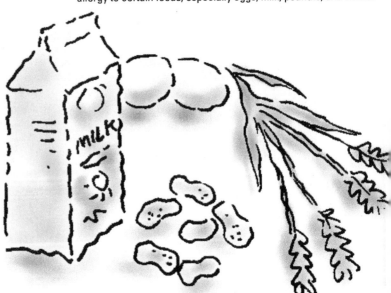

How it happens

In atopic dermatitis, the allergic mechanism of hypersensitivity results in a release of inflammatory mediators through sensitized antibodies of the IgE class. Histamine and other cytokines induce acute inflammation. Abnormally dry skin and a decreased threshold for itching set up the "itch-scratch-itch" cycle, which eventually causes lesions (excoriations, lichenification).

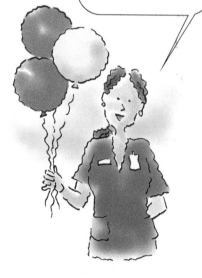

Risk factors for atopic dermatitis

- *Genetic factors*—greater chance of atopic dermatitis in children whose parents have allergic disorders
- *Environmental factors*—skin irritants, including wool or synthetic clothing, soaps or detergents, cosmetics or perfumes, dust and sand, chemical solvents, and chlorine; extremes in temperature or climate; and lack of moisturizing after bathing
- *Medical conditions*—allergies to plant pollen, animal dander, household dust mites, molds, and certain foods

A closer look

The top photo shows atopic dermatitis in an infant; the bottom one shows atopic dermatitis in an adult.

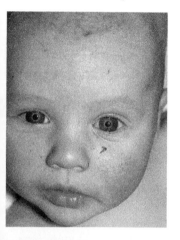

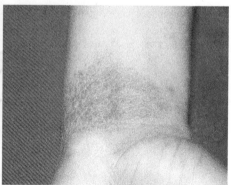

What to look for

- Erythematous, weeping lesions
- Scaling and lichenification of lesions
- In children: characteristic pink pigmentation and swelling of the upper eyelid and a double fold under the lower lid, called *Morgan line* or *Dennie sign*

These signs and symptoms make me think of yellow for weeping lesions, red for scaling lesions, and pink for pink pigmentation and swelling of the eyelids.

Rheumatoid arthritis

Rheumatoid arthritis (RA) is a chronic, systemic auto-immune, inflammatory disease that primarily attacks peripheral joints and the surrounding muscles, tendons, ligaments, and blood vessels. Partial remissions and unpredictable exacerbations mark the course of this potentially crippling disease.

RA is three times more common in women than men. It occurs worldwide, affecting more than 2.1 million people in the United States alone.

age-old story

Age and RA

RA can occur at any age, but the peak onset is ages 30 to 60. Women are more commonly affected than are men. Life expectancy for a person with RA may be shortened by an average of about 5 years.

How it happens

The cause of RA isn't known, but infections, genetics, environmental, and endocrine factors may play a part. When exposed to an unknown antigen, a person with RA shows activation of T cells and B cells in the joint regions. The B cells manufacture immunoglobulins (antibodies) that attack the joints causing synovitis (inflammation of the joint). These antibodies are sometimes detected as *rheumatoid factor* (*RF*) in the bloodstream. The activated T cells and B cells continually draw leukocytes to the joints, which secrete inflammatory mediators leading to cartilage damage. Immune responses continue, including complement system activation. Complement system activation attracts more leukocytes and stimulates the release of more inflammatory mediators, which then exacerbate joint destruction and form thick granulation tissue called a pannus.

Four stages of inflammation

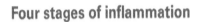

Stage 1

Synovitis develops from congestion and edema of the synovial membrane and joint capsule.

Stage 2

Formation of pannus (thickened layers of granulation tissue), which covers and invades cartilage and eventually destroys the joint capsule and bone.

Stage 3

Fibrous ankylosis (fibrous invasion of the pannus and scar formation that occludes the joint space) occurs. Bone atrophy and misalignment cause visible deformities and restrict movement, causing muscle atrophy, imbalance, and, possibly, partial dislocations.

Stage 4

Fibrous tissue calcifies, resulting in bony ankylosis (fixation of a joint) and total immobility. Pain associated with movement may restrict active joint use and cause fibrous or bony ankylosis, soft tissue contractures, and joint deformities.

Effects of RA on certain joints

Hand and wrist

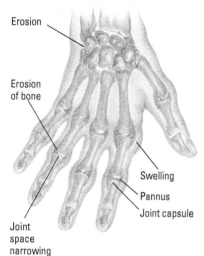

Erosion

Erosion of bone

Joint space narrowing

Swelling

Pannus

Joint capsule

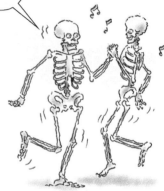

Ouch! These joints can't move like they used to!

Knee

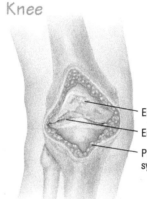

Erosion of cartilage

Erosion of bone

Pannus covering synovial membrane

memory board

Synovitis develops.

Pannus forms.

Ankylosis (fibrous) occurs.

Tissue calcifies.

My bones and brain are younger than yours.... So let's not have a SPAT.... Remember RA my way!

Hip

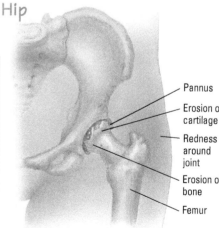

Pannus

Erosion of cartilage

Redness around joint

Erosion of bone

Femur

What to look for

* Fatigue
* Malaise
* Anorexia
* Persistent low-grade fever
* Weight loss
* Joint pains
* Joint stiffness (particularly in morning)
* Joint deformities (particularly of hands)

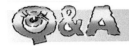

Photo finish

Number these illustrations (1 to 6) in the correct order as to how anaphylaxis develops.

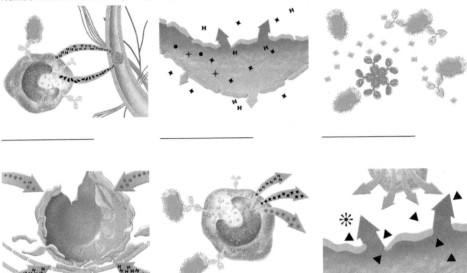

Riddle

Solve the riddle to learn a characteristic of a skin disorder.

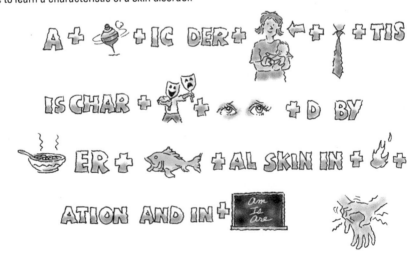

Selected References

Arnold, J. J., & Williams, P. M. (2011). Anaphylaxis: Recognition and management. *American Family Physician, 84*(10), 1111–1118.

Berke, R., Singh, A., & Guralnick, M. (2012). Atopic dermatitis: An overview. *American Family Physician, 86*(1) 35–42.

Braun, J., & Sieper, J. (2007). Ankylosing spondylitis. *Lancet, 369*(9570),1379–1390.

Chu, C., & Selwyn, P. A. (2011). Complications of HIV infection: A systems-based approach. *American Family Physician, 83*(4), 395–406.

Kumar, V., Abbas, A., & Aster, J. (2015). *Robbins and Cotran pathologic basis of disease* (9th ed.). Philadelphia, PA : Elsevier-Saunders.

Lee, K. C. (2014). Screening for HIV. *American Family Physician, 89*(8), 665–666.

Miossec, P. (2013). Rheumatoid arthritis: Still a chronic disease. *Lancet, 381*(9870), 84–86.

Saguil, A. (2013). Antiretroviral preexposure prophylaxis for preventing HIV infection in high-risk individuals. *American Family Physician, 88*(3), 172–173.

Scott, D. L., Wolfe, F., & Huizinga, T. W. (2010). Rheumatoid arthritis. *Lancet, 376*(9746), 1094–1108.

Sherin, K., Klekamp, B. G., Beal, J., & Martin, N. (2014). What is new in HIV infection? *American Family Physician, 89*(4), 265–272.

Sur, D. K., & Scandale, S. (2010). Treatment of allergic rhinitis. *American Family Physician, 81*(12), 1440–1446.

Chapter 9

Endocrine disorders

 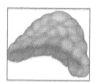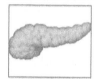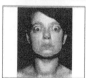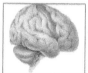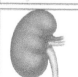
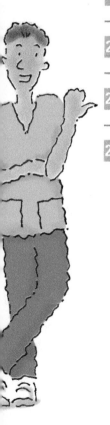

Adrenal hypofunction

Endocrine

Adrenal hypofunction occurs in two forms: primary and secondary. Both forms can progress into adrenal crisis.

Primary

Primary adrenal hypofunction or insufficiency (also called *Addison disease*) originates within the adrenal gland and is characterized by the decreased secretion of mineralocorticoids, glucocorticoids, and androgens. Addison disease is relatively uncommon and can occur at any age and in both genders.

Secondary

The secondary form of adrenal hypofunction is caused by a disorder outside the gland, such as a pituitary tumor with corticotropin deficiency, or abrupt withdrawal of long-term corticosteroid therapy. In secondary forms of the disorder, aldosterone secretion may be unaffected.

How it happens

In Addison disease, more than 90% of both adrenal glands are destroyed. Massive destruction usually results from an autoimmune process whereby circulating antibodies attack adrenal tissue. This leads to a rapid decline in the steroid hormones cortisol and aldosterone, which directly affects the liver, stomach, and kidneys.

Adrenal crisis

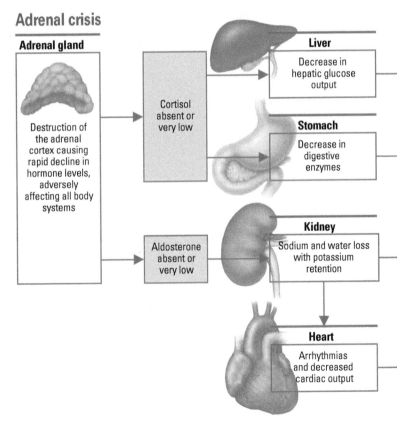

Adrenal gland

Destruction of the adrenal cortex causing rapid decline in hormone levels, adversely affecting all body systems

Cortisol absent or very low

Aldosterone absent or very low

Liver
Decrease in hepatic glucose output

Stomach
Decrease in digestive enzymes

Kidney
Sodium and water loss with potassium retention

Heart
Arrhythmias and decreased cardiac output

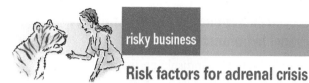

risky business

Risk factors for adrenal crisis

Adrenal crisis usually develops in patients who:
* Don't respond to hormone replacement therapy
* Experience extreme stress without adequate glucocorticoid replacement
* Abruptly stop hormone therapy
* Experience trauma
* Undergo bilateral adrenalectomy

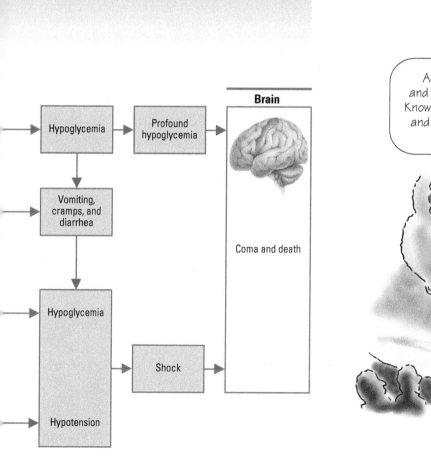

Blocked secretion of cortisol in primary adrenal hypofunction

Blocked secretion of cortisol in primary adrenal hypofunction results in feedback that causes hypersecretion of adrenocorticotropic hormone (ACTH) from the pituitary gland.

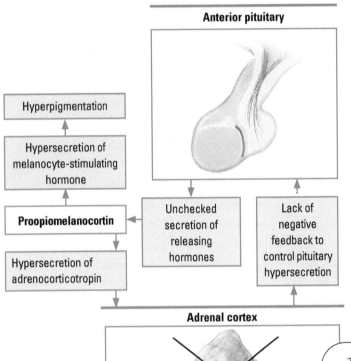

Anterior pituitary

Hyperpigmentation

Hypersecretion of melanocyte-stimulating hormone

Proopiomelanocortin

Hypersecretion of adrenocorticotropin

Unchecked secretion of releasing hormones

Lack of negative feedback to control pituitary hypersecretion

Adrenal cortex

Hypofunction of adrenal cortex, resulting in insufficient production of cortisol

What to look for

Primary
* Weakness and fatigue
* Weight loss, nausea, vomiting, and anorexia
* Conspicuous bronze color of the skin, especially in the creases of the hands and over the metacarpophalangeal joints (hand and finger), elbows, and knees
* Darkening of scars, areas of vitiligo (absence of pigmentation), and increased pigmentation of the mucous membranes, especially the buccal mucosa
* Orthostatic hypotension, decreased cardiac size and output, and weak, irregular pulse
* Decreased tolerance for even minor stress
* Fasting hypoglycemia
* Craving salty food

Secondary
* Similar to primary but without hyperpigmentation
* Possibly no hypotension and electrolyte abnormalities
* Usually normal androgen secretion

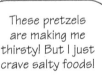

These pretzels are making me thirsty! But I just crave salty foods!

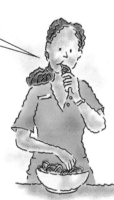

Diabetes mellitus

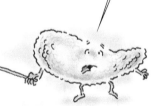

Diabetes mellitus occurs in two primary forms.

Diabetes mellitus is a disease in which the body doesn't produce or properly use insulin, leading to hyperglycemia.

> Type 1 diabetes: T1DM (due to absence of insulin from pancreas)

> Type 2 diabetes: T2DM (due to cellular insulin resistance) the more prevalent form

Several secondary forms also exist, caused by such conditions as pancreatic disease, pregnancy (gestational diabetes mellitus), hormonal or genetic problems, and certain drugs or chemicals.

How it happens

Normally, insulin allows glucose to travel into cells. There, it's used for energy and stored as glycogen. Insulin also stimulates protein synthesis and free fatty acid storage in adipose tissue. Insulin deficiency results in the inability of tissues to access essential nutrients for fuel and storage. The pathophysiology behind each type of diabetes differs.

Type 1 diabetes
* Pancreas makes no insulin.
* In genetically susceptible patients, an unknown triggering event (possibly a viral infection) causes production of autoantibodies against the beta cells of the pancreas.
* Resultant destruction of beta cells leads to ultimate lack of insulin secretion.
* Insulin deficiency leads to hyperglycemia with cell starvation. Cells go into starvation mode and start to breakdown body fat and muscle called lipolysis and protein catabolism.

Type 2 diabetes
* Genetic factors are significant.
* Onset is accelerated by obesity and a sedentary lifestyle.
* The pancreas produces some insulin, but it's either too little or ineffective.
* Cellular insulin resistance is the major cause.

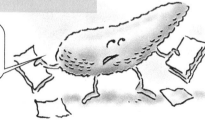

I have so many requests for insulin, I am exhausted !

Understanding type 2 diabetes

Normally, in response to blood glucose levels, the pancreatic islets of Langerhans release insulin. In type 2 diabetes, the body's cells resist insulin. With no cellular uptake of insulin, glucose builds up in the blood (hyperglycemia) and the pancreas keeps getting stimulated to secrete more insulin. Eventually, the pancreas is exhausted and has no insulin left.

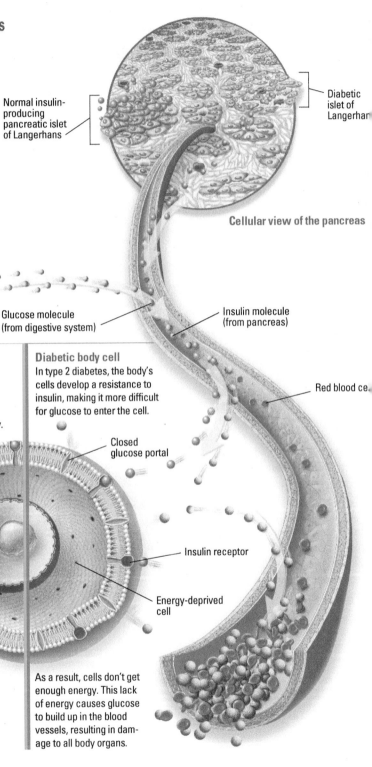

Normal insulin-producing pancreatic islet of Langerhans

Diabetic islet of Langerhans

Cellular view of the pancreas

Glucose molecule (from digestive system)

Insulin molecule (from pancreas)

Red blood cell

Normal body cell

Normally, insulin molecules bind to the preceptors on the body's cells. When activated by insulin, portals open to allow glucose to enter the cell, where it's converted to energy.

Diabetic body cell

In type 2 diabetes, the body's cells develop a resistance to insulin, making it more difficult for glucose to enter the cell.

Opened glucose portal

Closed glucose portal

Insulin receptor

Glucose converted to energy

Energy-deprived cell

As a result, cells don't get enough energy. This lack of energy causes glucose to build up in the blood vessels, resulting in damage to all body organs.

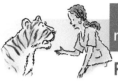

Risk factors for type 2 diabetes

- Older age
- Obesity
- Prediabetes also called glucose intolerance (blood glucose levels that are higher than normal but not yet high enough to be diagnosed as diabetes)
- Family history of diabetes
- Sedentary behavior
- Prior history of gestational diabetes
- Race or ethnicity (Blacks, Hispanics, and Native Americans)

memory board

Classic Symptom Triad in DM:

1-Polyuria (excessive urination)
2-Polydipsia (excessive thirst)
3-Polyphagia (excessive hunger)

Age and diabetes

Type 1 diabetes is the most common form of diabetes in children, but type 2 is on the rise owing to the obesity epidemic.

Diagnosis of diabetes is based on fasting blood glucose greater than 126 mg/dL or A1c level of greater than 6.5%.

I just can't get enough of this stuff!

What to look for

Type 1 diabetes
- Extreme thirst (polydipsia)
- High levels of ketones in urine
- Increase in appetite (polyphagia)
- Drowsiness and lethargy
- Fruity odor to breath
- Frequent urination (polyuria)
- High glucose levels in blood or urine
- Rapid, hard, or heavy breathing
- Eventual stupor to unconsciousness

Type 2 diabetes
- Possibly produces no symptoms
- Frequent urination (polyuria)
- Excessive thirst (polydipsia)
- Fatigue
- Very dry skin
- Sores that are slow to heal
- More infections than usual
- Dehydration
- Unexplained weight loss
- Extreme hunger (polyphagia)
- Sudden vision change

Hyperthyroidism

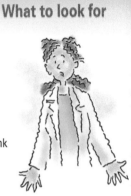

An overproduction of thyroid hormone creates a metabolic imbalance called *hyperthyroidism* or *thyrotoxicosis*. Excess thyroid hormone can cause various thyroid disorders; Graves disease is the most common.

How it happens

In Graves disease, thyroid-stimulating antibodies bind to and stimulate the thyroid-stimulating hormone (TSH) receptors of the thyroid gland.

The trigger for this autoimmune response is unclear; it may have several causes. Genetic factors may play a part because the disease tends to occur in identical twins. Immunologic factors may also be the culprit. The disease occasionally coexists with other autoimmune endocrine abnormalities, such as type 1 diabetes mellitus, thyroiditis, and hyperparathyroidism.

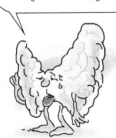

I feel grave. Actually, Graves disease is an autoimmune disorder that causes goiter and multiple systemic changes.

Anterior pituitary

↓

T-cell lymphocytes become sensitized to thyroid antigens.

↓

T-cell lymphocytes stimulate B-cell lymphocytes to secrete autoantibodies.

↓

Thyroid gland

Thyroid-stimulating antibodies bind to and stimulate TSH receptors of the thyroid gland.

↓

Increased production of thyroid hormones and cell growth result.

- With hyperthyroidism, a key to understanding the presentation is to think of hypermetabolism. Everything is on fast forward.
- Enlarged thyroid gland
- Exophthalmos (abnormal protrusion of the eye)
- Nervousness
- Heat intolerance
- Weight loss despite increased appetite
- Excessive sweating
- Diarrhea
- Tremors
- Palpitations

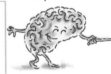

Central nervous system
- Difficulty concentrating
- Anxiety
- Excitability or nervousness, fine tremor, shaky handwriting, clumsiness, emotional instability, and mood swings ranging from occasional outbursts to overt psychosis

Cardiovascular system
- Most common in elderly patients
- Arrhythmias, especially atrial fibrillation
- Cardiac insufficiency
- Cardiac decompensation
- Resistance to the usual therapeutic dosage of digoxin

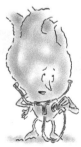

Integumentary system
- Vitiligo and skin hyperpigmentation
- Warm, moist, flushed skin with a velvety texture
- Fine, soft hair
- Premature graying
- Hair loss in both sexes
- Fragile nails
- Pretibial myxedema producing raised, thickened skin and plaquelike or nodular lesions on shins

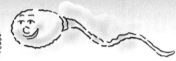

Reproductive system
- Menstrual abnormalities
- Impaired fertility
- Decreased libido
- Gynecomastia (abnormal development of mammary glands in men)

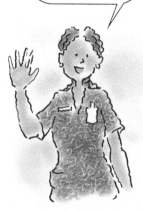

age-old story

Age and Graves disease

The incidence of Graves disease is greatest in women between ages 30 and 60, especially those with a family history of thyroid abnormalities.

Respiratory system
- Dyspnea on exertion and, possibly, at rest
- Breathlessness when climbing stairs

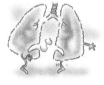

Eyes
- Infrequent blinking
- Lid lag
- Reddened conjunctiva and cornea
- Corneal ulcers
- Impaired upward gaze
- Convergence (turning the eyes in)
- Strabismus (eye deviation)
- Exophthalmos

GI system
- Anorexia
- Nausea and vomiting

Graves disease symptoms

This photo shows the major symptoms of Graves disease: exophthalmos and goiter.

Only 5% of patients with Graves disease are younger than age 15.

Musculoskeletal system
- Muscle weakness
- Generalized or localized muscle atrophy
- Osteoporosis

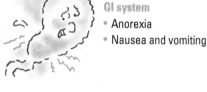

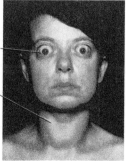

Exophthalmos

Goiter

Hypothyroidism

In hypothyroidism (thyroid hormone deficiency) in adults, metabolic processes slow down. This slowing is caused by a deficit in triiodothyronine (T_3) or thyroxine (T_4), both of which regulate metabolism.

Hypothyroidism is classified as *primary* or *secondary*. The primary form stems from a disorder of the thyroid gland itself. The secondary form stems from a failure of the pituitary gland to stimulate normal thyroid function.

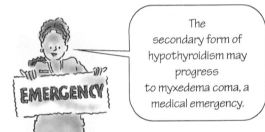

The secondary form of hypothyroidism may progress to myxedema coma, a medical emergency.

What to look for

- With hypothyroidism, a key to understanding the presentation is to think of hypometabolism. Everything slows down.

Early
- Energy loss
- Fatigue
- Forgetfulness
- Sensitivity to cold
- Unexplained weight gain
- Constipation

Progressive
- Anorexia
- Decreased libido
- Menorrhagia (excessive menstrual blood loss)
- Joint stiffness
- Muscle cramping

How it happens

Primary
- Thyroidectomy
- Inflammation from radiation therapy
- Other inflammatory conditions, such as amyloidosis and sarcoidosis
- Chronic autoimmune thyroiditis (Hashimoto disease)

Secondary
- Failure to stimulate normal thyroid function (e.g., the pituitary may fail to produce thyroid-stimulating hormone [TSH] [thyrotropin] or the hypothalamus may fail to produce thyrotropin-releasing hormone [TRH].)
- Inability to synthesize thyroid hormones due to iodine deficiency (usually dietary) or the use of antithyroid medications

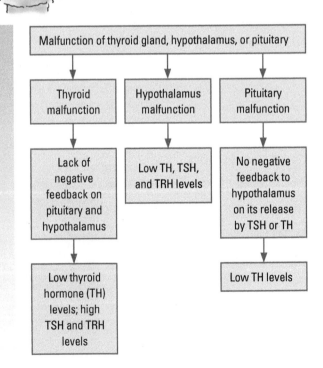

Malfunction of thyroid gland, hypothalamus, or pituitary

Thyroid malfunction	Hypothalamus malfunction	Pituitary malfunction
Lack of negative feedback on pituitary and hypothalamus	Low TH, TSH, and TRH levels	No negative feedback to hypothalamus on its release by TSH or TH
Low thyroid hormone (TH) levels; high TSH and TRH levels		Low TH levels

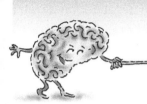

Central nervous system
- Psychiatric disturbances
- Ataxia (loss of coordination)
- Intention tremor (tremor during voluntary motion)
- Carpal tunnel syndrome
- Benign intracranial hypertension
- Behavioral changes ranging from slight mental slowing to severe impairment

Cardiovascular system
- Hypercholesterolemia (high cholesterol) with associated arteriosclerosis and ischemic heart disease
- Poor peripheral circulation
- Heart enlargement
- Heart failure
- Pleural and pericardial effusions

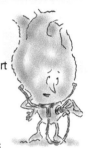

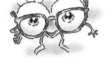

Eyes and ears
- Conductive or sensorineural deafness and nystagmus

GI system
- Achlorhydria (absence of free hydrochloric acid in the stomach)
- Pernicious anemia
- Adynamic (weak) colon, resulting in megacolon (extremely dilated colon) and intestinal obstruction

Integumentary system
- Dry, flaky, inelastic skin
- Puffy face, hands, and feet (called myxedema)
- Dry, sparse hair with patchy hair loss and loss of the outer third of the eyebrow
- Thick, brittle nails with transverse and longitudinal grooves
- Thick, dry tongue, causing hoarseness and slow, slurred speech

Reproductive system
- Impaired fertility

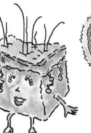

Hematologic system
- Anemia, possibly resulting in bleeding tendencies and iron deficiency anemia

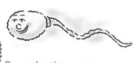

age-old story

Age and hypothyroidism

Hypothyroidism occurs primarily after age 40. In fact, 10% of all women older than age 50 show signs of a failing thyroid, as opposed to 3% of men older than age 50.

Myxedema coma is a life-threatening condition, which represents a form of decompensated hypothyroidism in patients with long-standing, severe untreated hypothyroidism. Patients with myxedema coma present with altered mental status (disorientation, lethargy, psychosis, or coma), defects in thermoregulation (hypothermia or absence of fever during an infection), and onset of symptoms due to a precipitating stressor (trauma, infection, cold exposure, stroke, heart failure, or GI bleed). Altered body temperature results in diminished energy production, decreased cardiac function, and pulmonary failure.

Metabolic syndrome

Metabolic syndrome is a cluster of conditions characterized by:
- Abdominal obesity
- High blood glucose level (type 2 diabetes mellitus)
- Insulin resistance
- High blood cholesterol and triglyceride levels
- High blood pressure
  More than 22% of people in the United States demonstrate three or more of these characteristics, meeting the requirements for a diagnosis of metabolic syndrome.

  Diagnosis of metabolic syndrome has a relative risk of approximately twofold for cardiovascular disease over 5 to 10 years and at least fivefold for type 2 diabetes.

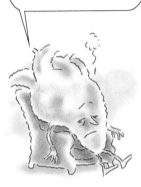

Metabolic syndrome raises a person's risk of heart disease and stroke and places him or her at high risk for dying of a myocardial infarction.

How it happens

In the normal digestion process, the intestines break down food into its basic components, one of which is glucose. Glucose provides energy for cellular activity, and excess glucose is stored in cells for future use. Insulin, a hormone secreted in the pancreas, transports glucose into cells for metabolism or storage.

However, in people with metabolic syndrome, cells in the body have a diminished ability to respond to insulin or they are "insulin resistant" and they do not respond to insulin's attempt to transport glucose into cells. Excess insulin is needed to overcome resistance which increases fat deposits. Excess glucose remains in the blood and causes damage to the lining of the arteries leading to cardiovascular disease.

Effects of metabolic syndrome

Organs affected by metabolic syndrome

Brain	Pancreas	Heart
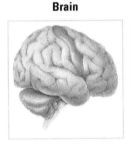	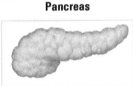	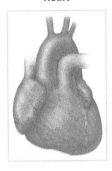

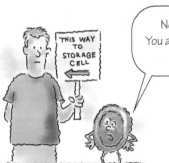

No way, man. You aren't the boss of me!

THIS WAY TO STORAGE CELL

Fibrous plaque (atherosclerosis)

What to look for

> Symptom: abdominal obesity (evidenced by a waist of more than 40 [101.6 cm] in men and 35 [88.9 cm] in women) caused by poor diet and sedentary lifestyle

> Symptom: blood pressure of 130/85 mm Hg or higher due to a history of hypertension

> Symptom: fasting blood glucose level of 100 mg/dL or higher due to diabetes or prediabetes

High blood glucose
Glucose builds up in the bloodstream.

High blood pressure
If untreated, damage to the lining of the arteries results.

Fibrous plaque
Elevated cholesterol levels lead to fibrous deposits in the blood vessels.

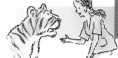

risky business

Risk factors for metabolic syndrome

The American Heart Association has determined that a patient with three or more of these factors is at risk for developing metabolic syndrome:

• Elevated waist circumference—40' (101.6 cm) or more in men; 35' (88.9 cm) or more in women
• Elevated triglyceride level—150 mg/dL or higher
• Reduced HDL ("good") cholesterol—less than 40 mg/dL in men; less than 50 mg/dL in women
• Elevated blood pressure—130/85 mm Hg or higher
• Elevated fasting glucose level—100 mg/dL or higher

SIADH

The syndrome of inappropriate antidiuretic hormone secretion (SIADH) results when excessive antidiuretic hormone (ADH) secretion is triggered by stimuli other than increased extracellular fluid osmolarity and decreased extracellular fluid volume. SIADH is a relatively common complication of surgery or critical illness—most commonly brain surgery, lung cancer, or other disease of the CNS. It may develop in some children during the acute phase of meningitis. The prognosis varies with the degree of disease and the speed at which it develops. SIADH usually resolves within 3 days of effective treatment.

What to look for

- Fatigue, lethargy, and anorexia
- Vomiting
- Intestinal cramping
- Weight gain
- Edema
- Water retention
- Decreased urine output
- Restlessness
- Confusion
- Headache
- Irritability
- Seizures
- Coma
- Decreased deep tendon reflexes

How it happens

In the presence of excessive ADH, excessive water from the distal tubule and collecting ducts of the nephron is reabsorbed into the bloodstream, which causes dilutional hyponatremia and increased extracellular fluid volume.

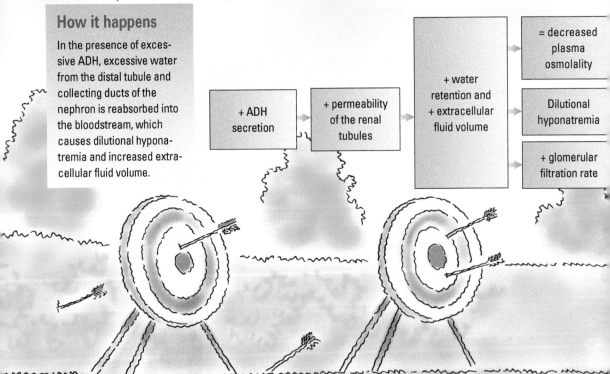

+ ADH secretion → + permeability of the renal tubules → + water retention and + extracellular fluid volume → = decreased plasma osmolality

Dilutional hyponatremia

+ glomerular filtration rate

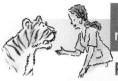

Risk factors for SIADH

- Recent surgery or critical illness
- Oat cell or small cell lung cancer (secretes excessive ADH), pancreatic or prostate cancer
- Hodgkin disease
- Central nervous system disorders
- Pulmonary disorders
- Certain drugs
- Myxedema
- Psychosis

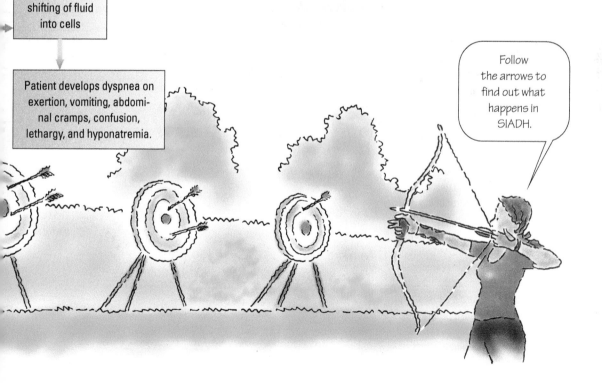

+ sodium excretion and a shifting of fluid into cells

Patient develops dyspnea on exertion, vomiting, abdominal cramps, confusion, lethargy, and hyponatremia.

Follow the arrows to find out what happens in SIADH.

Thyroid cancer

Thyroid cancer (also called *thyroid carcinoma*) is the most common endocrine malignancy. It occurs in all age groups, especially in people who have undergone radiation treatment of the neck area. There are three main types:

Papillary

Follicular

Medullary

How it happens

Papillary carcinoma accounts for one-half of all thyroid cancers in adults. Most common in young females, it's the least virulent form of thyroid cancer and metastasizes slowly.

Follicular carcinoma is less common but more likely to recur and metastasize to the regional lymph nodes and through blood vessels into the bones, liver, and lungs.

Medullary carcinoma originates in the parafollicular cells and contains amyloid and calcium deposits. It can produce thyrocalcitonin, histamine, adrenocorticotropin (producing Cushing syndrome), and prostaglandins E_2 and F_3 (producing diarrhea). This rare form of thyroid cancer is familial, associated with pheochromocytoma, and completely curable when detected before it causes symptoms. Untreated, it progresses rapidly. Seldom curable by resection, these tumors resist radiation and metastasize quickly.

Early, localized thyroid cancer

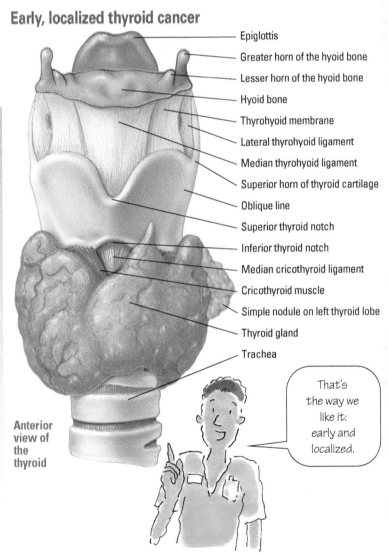

- Epiglottis
- Greater horn of the hyoid bone
- Lesser horn of the hyoid bone
- Hyoid bone
- Thyrohyoid membrane
- Lateral thyrohyoid ligament
- Median thyrohyoid ligament
- Superior horn of thyroid cartilage
- Oblique line
- Superior thyroid notch
- Inferior thyroid notch
- Median cricothyroid ligament
- Cricothyroid muscle
- Simple nodule on left thyroid lobe
- Thyroid gland
- Trachea

Anterior view of the thyroid

That's the way we like it: early and localized.

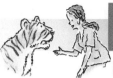

Risk factors for thyroid cancer

- Age older than 40
- Gender (three times more common in women than in men)
- Race (more common in Whites than Blacks)
- Iodine deficiency
- Radiation exposure
- High-dose x-rays to neck region
- Heredity (family history of thyroid cancer, goiter, or colon polyps)
- Thyroid cancer has been projected to be the fourth leading cancer diagnosis by 2030.

Papillary carcinoma of the thyroid

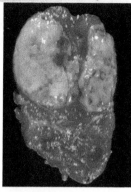

This photograph shows a resected thyroid gland with a beige mass, which is papillary carcinoma.

Follicular adenoma

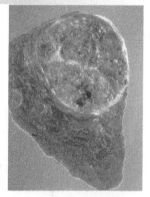

This photograph shows an encapsulated mass of follicular adenoma with hemorrhage, fibrosis, and cystic changes.

Medullary thyroid carcinoma

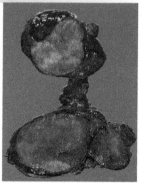

This photograph shows a section of a thyroid resection with a pale tumor, indicating medullary carcinoma.

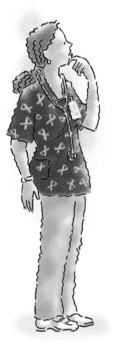

What to look for

- Painless nodule, hard nodule in an enlarged thyroid gland, or palpable lymph nodes and thyroid enlargement
- Cough
- Hoarseness, dysphagia, and pain on palpation
- Hypothyroidism (low metabolism, mental apathy, sensitivity to cold) or hyperthyroidism (hyperactivity, restlessness, sensitivity to heat)
- Diarrhea, anorexia, irritability, and vocal cord paralysis

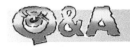

My word!

Solve the word scrambles to discover four major signs and symptoms of diabetes mellitus. Then, rearrange the circled letters from those words to answer the question posed.

Show and tell

Identify the two signs of Graves disease pictured in this photo and explain their importance.

Question: What is a major component of diabetes mellitus?

1. remxtee stthri — — — — — — —   — —◯—◯—

2. gutifae — — — — —◯—

3. reqenutf naonruiti — — — — — —◯—   — — — — — — — —◯

4. redltae ppttaeie —◯— — — — —   — — — — —◯— —

Answer: — — — — — —

1. _____
_____
_____
_____

2. _____
_____
_____
_____

Selected References

Bassi, N., Karagodin, I., Wang, S., Vassallo, P., Priyanath, A., Massaro, E., & Stone N. J. (2014). Lifestyle modification for metabolic syndrome: A systematic review. *American Journal of Medicine, 127*(12), 1242.e1–1242.e10.

Cohen, D. M., & Ellison, D. H. (2015). Evaluating hyponatremia. *Journal of the American Medical Association, 313*(12), 1260–1261.

George, C. M., Brujin, L. L., Will, K., & Howard-Thompson, A.(2015). Management of blood glucose with noninsulin therapies in type 2 diabetes. *American Family Physician, 92*(1), 27–34.

Keeble, D. S., Farland, M. Z., & Eaddy, J. (2014). Glycemic control is an important consideration in diabetes care. *American Family Physician, 90*(8), 524–526.

Knox, M. A. (2013). Thyroid nodules. *American Family Physician, 88*(3), 193–196.

Liao, E. P. (2012). Management of type 2 diabetes: New and future developments in treatment. *American Journal of Medicine, 125*(10), S2–S3.

Michels, A., & Michels, N. (2014). Addison disease: Early detection and treatment principles. *American Family Physician, 89*(7), 563–568.

Morley, J. E. (2015). Dehydration, hypernatremia, and hyponatremia. *Clinical Geriatric Medicine, 31*(3), 389–399.

Pluta, R. M., Burke, A. E., & Golub, R. M. (2011). JAMA patient page. Cushing syndrome and Cushing disease. *Journal of the American Medical Association, 306*(24), 2742.

Pratley, R. E., Kuritzky, L., & Tenzer, P. (2014). A patient-centered approach to managing patients with type 2 diabetes. *American Journal of Medicine, 127*(11), e15–e16.

Chapter 10

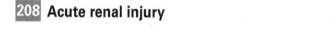

Kidney and urological disorders

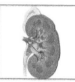

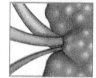

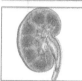

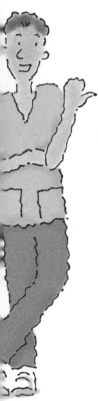

Acute renal injury

Renal

Acute renal injury is the sudden interruption of renal function. It can be caused by obstruction, poor circulation, or kidney disease. It's potentially reversible; however, if left untreated, permanent damage can lead to chronic renal failure.

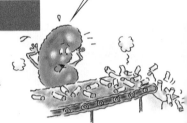

Oh no! An interruption in my work flow! This can lead to serious failure!

How it happens

Acute renal injury may be classified as prerenal, intrarenal, or postrenal. Each type has separate causes.

Mechanism of acute renal injury

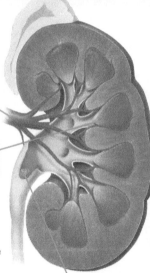

Prerenal injury
(any cause of marked decrease in renal blood flow)

- Antihypertensives (if they lower BP too much)
- Arrhythmias that cause reduced cardiac output
- Arterial embolism (that causes decreased circulation to kidney)
- Arterial or venous thrombosis (that causes decreased circulation to kidney)
- Burns
- Cardiac tamponade
- Cardiogenic shock
- Severe dehydration
- Diuretic overuse (that causes decreased BP)
- Heart failure (that causes decreased BP)
- Hemorrhage
- Hypovolemic shock
- Malignant hypertension
- Myocardial infarction (that causes decreased BP)
- Trauma (which causes hemorrhage)
- Vasculitis

Intrarenal injury
(any etiology that damages structures of the kidney)

- Acute glomerulonephritis
- Acute tubular necrosis
- Acute pyelonephritis
- Crush injuries
- Malignant nephrosclerosis
- Myopathy (causing excessive myoglobinuria, which can clog nephrons)
- Nephrotoxins (e.g., drugs such as aminoglycoside antibiotics)
- Papillary necrosis
- Scleroderma of kidney
- Systemic lupus erythematosus
- Transfusion reaction
- Vasculitis of kidney

Postrenal injury
(any cause of obstruction of urine outflow from kidney)

- Kidney stone
- Bladder obstruction
- Benign prostatic hyperplasia
- Prostate cancer
- Malignancy of urologic syste
- Ureteral obstruction
- Urethral obstruction

Phases of acute renal injury

The three types of acute renal injury (prerenal, intrarenal, and postrenal) usually include three distinct phases: oliguric, diuretic, and recovery.

Oliguric phase

Decreased urine output of less than 400 mL/24 hours (oliguria)

▼

Decreased blood flow to the kidney (prerenal oliguria)

▼

Impairment of kidney's ability to conserve sodium

▼

Acute tubular necrosis possibly resulting from prerenal oliguria

▼

Increased blood urea nitrogen (BUN) and creatinine levels and decreased ratio of BUN to creatinine (from normal levels of 20:1 to abnormal decrease of 10:1)

▼

Hypervolemia

▼

Edema, weight gain, and elevated blood pressure

Diuretic phase

Slow increase in BUN and creatinine levels

▼

Hypovolemia and weight loss

▼

Decreased potassium, sodium, and water levels

▼

Death if untreated

Recovery phase

Normal BUN and creatinine levels with urine output between 1 and 2 L/day

What to look for

Acute renal injury is a critical illness. Its early signs and symptoms are oliguria (decreased urine output to <400 mL/day), azotemia (excess levels of urea nitrogen in blood), high serum creatinine, and edema. Electrolyte imbalances such as hyperkalemia, hypocalcemia, hyperphosphatemia, and metabolic acidosis occur as the patient becomes increasingly uremic and renal dysfunction disrupts other body systems. Red blood cells and platelets lyse due to high nitrogen in the blood causing anemia and thrombocytopenia (lack of clotting ability). The brain cannot function properly with high nitrogen in the blood; the condition is called uremic encephalopathy. Erythropoietin is not secreted by a damaged kidney, causing anemia. Renin is oversecreted by a damaged kidney, causing hypertension.

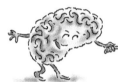

Central nervous system (called uremic encephalopathy)
- Headache
- Drowsiness
- Irritability
- Confusion
- Peripheral neuropathy (burning and pruritus)
- Seizures
- Coma

GI system
- Anorexia
- Nausea and vomiting
- Bleeding (due to low platelets)
- Dry mucous membranes
- Uremic breath

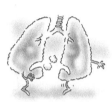

Respiratory system
- Pulmonary edema
- Kussmaul respirations

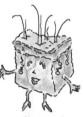

Integumentary system
- Dry skin
- Pruritus
- Pallor (due to anemia)
- Purpura

Cardiovascular system
- Hypertension
- Arrhythmia
- Fluid overload
- Heart failure
- Systemic edema
- Anemia (RBC lysis in high nitrogen blood and lack of erythropoietin)
- Altered clotting mechanisms; low platelets

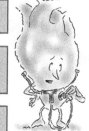

Acute tubular necrosis

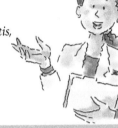

ATN causes 75% of all cases of acute renal injury.

Acute tubular necrosis (ATN), also called *acute tubulointerstitial nephritis*, destroys the tubular segment of the nephron, causing uremia (excess accumulation of nitrogen from protein breakdown in blood) and renal injury.

How it happens

ATN results from ischemic or nephrotoxic injury, most commonly in debilitated patients, such as the critically ill and those who have undergone extensive surgery.

In ischemic injury, disruption of blood flow to the kidneys may result from circulatory collapse, severe hypotension, trauma, hemorrhage, dehydration, cardiogenic or septic shock, surgery, anesthetics, or reactions to transfusions. Ischemic ATN can damage the epithelial and basement membranes and cause lesions in the renal interstitium and is, therefore, irreversible.

Nephrotoxic injury may result from ingestion of certain chemical agents (such as contrast media administered during radiologic procedures), administration of antibiotics (aminoglycosides), or a hypersensitive reaction of the kidneys. Because nephrotoxic ATN doesn't damage the basement membrane of the nephron, it's potentially reversible.

Ischemic necrosis

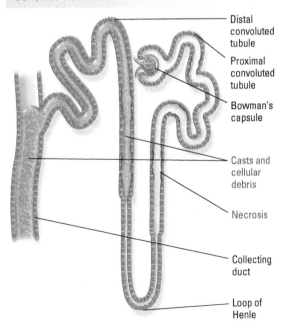

- Distal convoluted tubule
- Proximal convoluted tubule
- Bowman's capsule
- Casts and cellular debris
- Necrosis
- Collecting duct
- Loop of Henle

Nephrotoxic injury

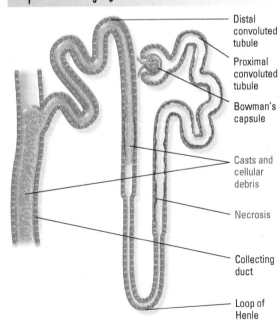

- Distal convoluted tubule
- Proximal convoluted tubule
- Bowman's capsule
- Casts and cellular debris
- Necrosis
- Collecting duct
- Loop of Henle

What to look for

- Decreased urine output
- Hyperkalemia
- Uremic syndrome with oliguria (or, rarely, anuria) and confusion, which may progress to uremic coma
- Dry mucous membranes and skin
- Alteration in level of consciousness
- Central nervous system signs and symptoms, such as lethargy, twitching, and seizures

> ATN is usually difficult to recognize in its early stages because effects of the critically ill patient's primary disease may mask ATN's symptoms.

Pathogenesis of acute tubular necrosis

In ATN, the tubules of the nephrons undergo ischemia and become necrotic. The necrotic tubule epithelial cells slough off and cause obstruction within the lumens of the tubules. This causes an increase in the intraluminal pressure of the tubules causing decreased glomerular filtration. Increased intraluminal pressure causes fluid to leak into the interstitium of the kidney. Sloughed tubule epithelial cells are excreted as casts in the urine.

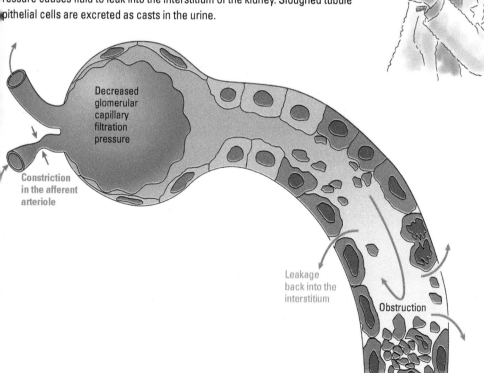

Decreased glomerular capillary filtration pressure

Constriction in the afferent arteriole

Leakage back into the interstitium

Obstruction

Glomerulonephritis

Glomerulonephritis is a bilateral inflammation of the glomeruli that follows a streptococcal infection in certain susceptible individuals.

How it happens

Acute poststreptococcal glomerulonephritis results from an immune response that occurs in the glomerulus. A streptococcal infection of the throat usually begins the process. The antibodies that the body forms against the streptococcal organisms attack the glomeruli membranes and cause inflammation. Glomerular injury occurs as a result of the inflammatory process. Glomerular injury causes increased permeability of the glomerular capillaries and proteins, and RBCs seep out of the capillary blood into the tubule fluid, which becomes urine. As proteins are lost from the blood, colloid oncotic pressure decreases and edema results. Proteinuria, hematuria, and edema are key signs of glomerulonephritis. Hypertension also occurs due to high renin secretion in kidney injury.

We're the antigen gang, known as group A beta-hemolytic streptococci. We'll be first to respond to any disturbance!

When someone tries to change us, we stimulate antibody formation.

Acute poststreptococcal glomerulonephritis

Yeah, lodge it into the glomerular capillaries!

I bet that'll cause an inflammatory response!

This inflammatory process has the antigen-antibody complexes initiating the release of inflammatory mediators!

Don't look now, but I think those inflammatory mediators are going to wear us down and increase membrane permeability!

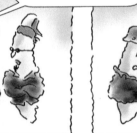

Glomerular injury

Age and glomerulonephritis

In children, the characteristic features of glomeru-lonephritis are hypertension, proteinuria, hematuria, and periorbital edema.

An elderly patient with glomerulonephritis may report vague, nonspecific symptoms, such as nausea, malaise, dark urine, hypertension, edema, and arthralgia.

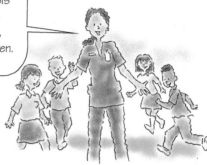

To prevent glomerulonephritis, it is important to get early diagnosis and treatment of strep throat, especially in children.

Immune complex deposits on the glomerulus

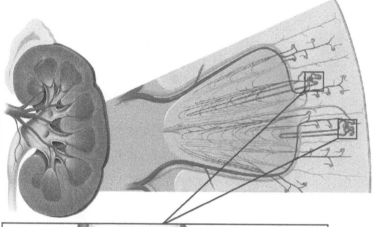

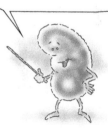

The severity of glomerular damage and renal insufficiency is related to the size, number, location, duration of exposure, and type of antigen-antibody complexes.

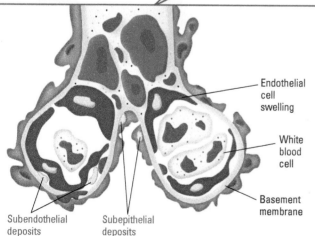

Endothelial cell swelling

White blood cell

Basement membrane

Subendothelial deposits

Subepithelial deposits

What to look for

- Decreased urination or oliguria
- Dark urine (hematuria)
- Shortness of breath
- Periorbital edema
- Edema of the lower extremities
- Edema of the abdomen
- Foamy urine (due to proteinuria)
- Mild to severe hypertension
- Nausea
- Malaise
- Arthralgia

Hydronephrosis

An abnormal dilation of the renal pelvis and the calyces of one or both kidneys, hydronephrosis is caused by an obstruction of urine flow in the genitourinary tract.

> Almost any type of disease that results from obstruction of the urinary tract can result in hydronephrosis.

How it happens

If the obstruction is in the urethra or bladder, hydronephrosis usually affects both kidneys. If the obstruction is in a ureter, it usually affects one kidney. Obstructions distal to the bladder cause the bladder to dilate and act as a buffer zone, delaying hydronephrosis. Total obstruction of urine flow with dilation of the collecting system ultimately causes complete atrophy of the cortex (the outer portion of the kidney) and cessation of glomerular filtration. Potential causes include congenital abnormalities, scar tissue from previous injuries or surgery, kinking of the ureter, persistent kidney stones, tumors, pregnancy, or inflammatory conditions of the urinary tract that cause obstructed urine outflow.

Renal damage in hydronephrosis

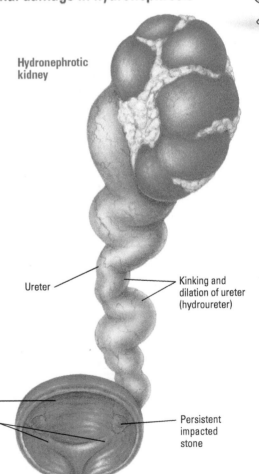

Hydronephrotic kidney

Ureter

Kinking and dilation of ureter (hydroureter)

Bladder

Ureteral openings

Persistent impacted stone

A closer look

This photograph shows dilation of the ureters, renal pelvises, and renal calyces from bilateral urinary tract obstruction.

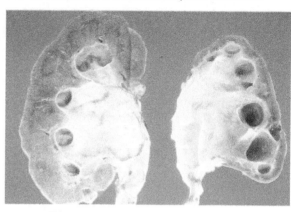

Dilated calyces

Cross section of hydronephrotic kidney

Atrophied parenchyma and tubules

Atrophied papilla

Dilated pelvis

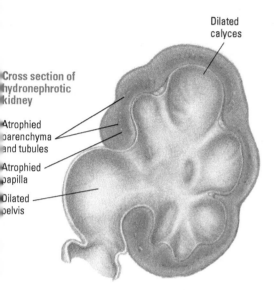

Signs and symptoms of hydronephrosis depend on the cause of the obstruction.

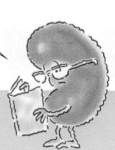

What to look for

Mild
* No symptoms
* Mild pain—may be of flank, abdomen, or groin
* Slightly decreased urine flow

Severe
* Severe, colicky renal pain or dull flank pain
* Hematuria
* Pyuria (white blood cells in urine)
* Dysuria
* Alternating polyuria and oliguria, and complete anuria

General
* Nausea and vomiting
* Abdominal fullness
* Dribbling of urine
* Urinary hesitancy

Polycystic kidney disease

Polycystic kidney disease (PKD) is an inherited disorder characterized by multiple, bilateral, grapelike clusters of fluid-filled cysts that enlarge the kidneys, compressing and eventually replacing functioning renal tissue. The disease affects males and females equally and appears in three distinct forms.

Autosomal dominant polycystic kidney disease (ADPKD) is the most common type and accounts for about 10% of all cases of end-stage renal disease in the United States.

Another inherited form is called *autosomal recessive PKD*. It's a rare form that can exhibit symptoms when a fetus is still in the womb.

Acquired cystic kidney disease is the third form. This form isn't inherited and tends to occur in the later stages of life. It's associated with long-term kidney problems, especially kidney failure, and is prevalent in patients who have been receiving dialysis for a long period of time.

How it happens

Multiple spherical cysts, a few millimeters to centimeters in diameter, containing straw-colored or hemorrhagic fluid, cause grossly enlarged kidneys. The cysts are distributed evenly throughout the cortex and medulla. Renal parenchyma may have varying degrees of tubular atrophy, interstitial fibrosis, and nephrosclerosis. The cysts cause elongation of the renal pelvis, flattening of the calyces, and indentations in the kidney.

Commonly, a syndrome exists of intracranial aneurysms, colonic diverticula, and mitral valve prolapse. Cysts develop in other organs as well.

> In most cases, progressive compression of kidney structures by the enlarging mass causes renal failure about 10 years after symptoms appear.

> With polycystic kidney disease, I won't look this healthy for long. Cysts can develop on the liver, spleen, pancreas, and ovaries.

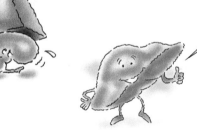

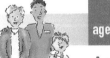

age-old story

Age and polycystic kidney disease

Renal deterioration is more gradual in adults than infants. However, in both age-groups, the disease progresses relentlessly to fatal uremia.

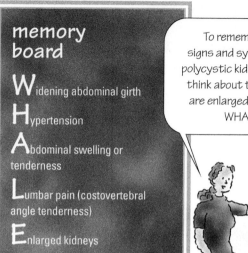

memory board

Widening abdominal girth

Hypertension

Abdominal swelling or tenderness

Lumbar pain (costovertebral angle tenderness)

Enlarged kidneys

To remember the signs and symptoms of polycystic kidney disease, think about things that are enlarged, such as a WHALE!

What to look for

- Hypertension
- Lumbar pain (classic kidney pain occurs in the costovertebral angle of lumbar region)
- Widening abdominal girth
- Swollen or tender abdomen
- Grossly enlarged kidneys on palpation
- Polyuria
- Hematuria
- Recurrent urinary tract infections

Polycystic kidney

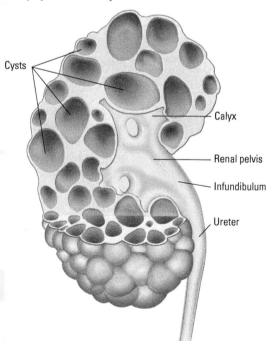

Cysts

Calyx

Renal pelvis

Infundibulum

Ureter

Adult polycystic disease

This photograph shows the enlarged, polycystic kidney of an adult (whole kidney on the left; cross section on the right). Note that cysts have taken the place of almost all of the parenchyma.

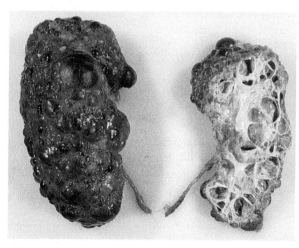

Pyelonephritis

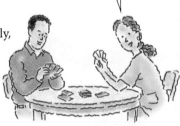

Chances are, I'll get pyelonephritis before he does!

Acute pyelonephritis is a sudden inflammation caused by bacteria that primarily affects the interstitial area and the renal pelvis or, less commonly, the renal tubules. It's one of the most common renal diseases and may affect one or both kidneys. With treatment and continued follow-up care, the prognosis is good, and extensive permanent damage is rare.

Pyelonephritis is more common in females, probably because of the shorter female urethra and the proximity of the urinary meatus to the vagina and the rectum. Both conditions allow bacteria to reach the bladder more easily. In males, pyelonephritis may occur due to a lack of the antibacterial prostatic secretions normally produced in males or due to prostate enlargement that obstructs urine outflow.

How it happens

Typically, the infection spreads from the bladder to the ureters and then to the kidneys, as in vesicoureteral reflux. Vesico-ureteral reflux may result from congenital weakness at the junction of the ureter and the bladder. Bacteria refluxed to intrarenal tissues may create colonies of infection within 24 to 48 hours. Infection may also result from instrumentation (such as catheterization, cys-toscopy, or urologic surgery), from a hematogenic infection (as in septicemia or endocar-ditis), or, possibly, from lym-phatic infection.

Pyelonephritis may also result from an inability to empty the bladder (for exam-ple, in patients with neuro-genic bladder), urinary stasis, or urinary obstruction due to tumors, strictures, or benign prostatic hyperplasia.

Phases of pyelonephritis

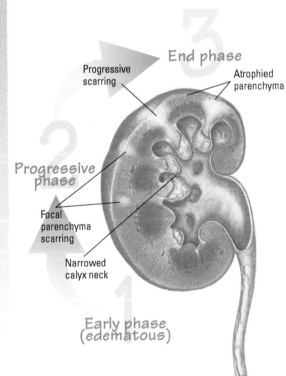

End phase

Progressive scarring

Atrophied parenchyma

Progressive phase

Focal parenchyma scarring

Narrowed calyx neck

Early phase (edematous)

age-old story

Age and pyelonephritis

Elderly patients may exhibit GI symptoms or confusion and disorientation rather than the usual febrile responses to pyelonephritis. Elderly adults do not run a fever—infection in an elderly adult more com-monly causes behavioral changes. In younger adults, fever, chills, hematuria, and flank pain are common. In children younger than age 2, fever, vomiting, nonspecific abdominal com-plaints, and failure to thrive may be the only signs of acute pyelonephritis.

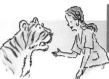

risky business

Risk factors for pyelonephritis

Incidence of pyelonephritis increases with age and is higher in the following groups:
* *Sexually active women*—Intercourse increases the risk of bacterial contamination of the urinary tract.
* *Pregnancy*—About 5% develop bacteriuria that produces no symptoms; if untreated, about 40% develop pyelonephritis.
* *Diabetes*—Neurogenic bladder causes incomplete emptying and urinary stasis; glycosuria increases risk of bacterial growth in the urine.
* *People with other renal diseases*—Compromised renal function aggravates susceptibility.

What to look for
* Urinary urgency and frequency, burning during urination, dysuria, nocturia, and hematuria
* Cloudy urine that has an ammonia-like or fishy odor
* Temperature of 102°F (38.9°C) or higher, shaking chills, nausea and vomiting, flank pain, anorexia, and general fatigue

A look at chronic pyelonephritis

These photographs show the effects of chronic pyelonephritis on the kidneys.

In the first photo, you can see many reddish areas that indicate scarring. In the second photo, you can see severe dilation of the calyces as well as atrophy and scarring of the cortex.

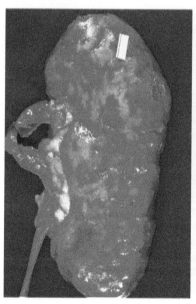
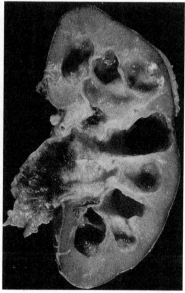

Renal calculi

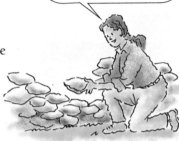

Some say good fences make good neighbors, but this many stones spells trouble for kidneys!

Also called *nephrolithiasis*, renal calculi (stones) can form anywhere in the urinary tract, although they most commonly develop in the renal pelvis or calyx. They may vary in size and may be solitary or multiple.

The major types of renal calculi are calcium oxalate and calcium phosphate, accounting for 75% to 80% of calculi. Struvite (magnesium, ammonium, and phosphate) accounts for 15%; uric acid, 7%.

How it happens

Nephrolithiasis occurs in susceptible individuals due to genetics, elevated mineral content of the blood, and dehydration. Calculi form when substances that are normally dissolved in the urine, such as calcium oxalate and calcium phosphate, precipitate out into the urine. Dehydration often leads to renal calculi as calculus-forming substances become concentrated in the urine.

Finish

Calculi may occur in the papillae, renal tubules, calyces, renal pelvis, ureter, or bladder. Many calculi are less than 5 mm in diameter and are usually passed in the urine.

Staghorn calculi can continue to grow in the pelvis and extend to the calyces, forming a branching calculus and, ultimately, resulting in renal failure if not surgically removed.

Calculi may be composed of different substances, and the pH of the urine affects the solubility of many calculus-forming substances.

A crystal evolves in the presence of calculus-forming substances (calcium oxalate, calcium carbonate, magnesium, ammonium, phosphate, or uric acid) and becomes trapped in the urinary tract, where it attracts other crystals to form a calculus.

A high urine saturation of these substances encourages crystal formation and results in calculus growth.

Hop along with me and see how it all happens!

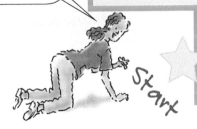

Start

Calculi form around a nidus in the appropriate environment.

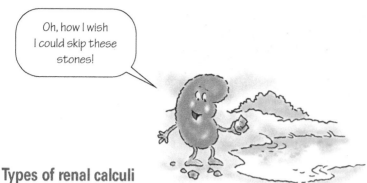

Oh, how I wish I could skip these stones!

Types of renal calculi

Uric acid stones

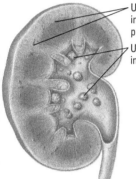

Urate deposits in renal parenchyma

Urate stones in pelvis

Ammoniomagnesium phosphate (struvite) stones

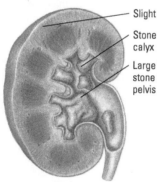

Slight renal edema

Stone forming in calyx

Large "staghorn" stone in renal pelvis

A look at staghorn calculi

This photo shows a kidney with hydronephrosis and staghorn calculi, which are casts of the dilated calyces.

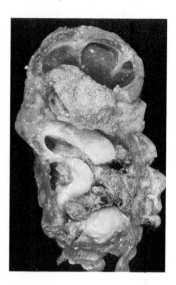

Calcium stones

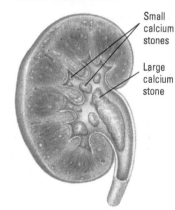

Small calcium stones

Large calcium stone

What to look for

- Pain resulting from obstruction (possibly mild to severe deep flank pain or tenderness or abrupt, severe, colicky flank pain)
- Nausea and vomiting
- Fever and chills (from infection)
- Hematuria (when calculi abrade a ureter)
- Urinary hesitancy and dysuria (due to obstruction)
- Abdominal distention
- Anuria (from bilateral obstruction or obstruction of a patient's only kidney)

Renovascular hypertension

Renovascular hypertension occurs when systemic blood pressure increases due to intrarenal atherosclerosis or stenosis of the major renal arteries or their branches. This narrowing (also called stenosis) may be partial or complete, and the resulting blood pressure elevation may be benign or malignant. Renovascular hypertension is the most common type of secondary hypertension.

> I can just feel the renin risin'. Nobody knows the trouble I've seen...

How it happens

The kidneys normally play a key role in maintaining blood pressure and volume by vasoconstriction and regulation of sodium and fluid levels. In renovascular hypertension, these regulatory mechanisms fail.

1 Certain conditions, such as renal artery stenosis, reduce blood flow to the kidneys. This reduced flow causes juxtaglomerular cells to continuously secrete renin.

In this stage, be alert for flank pain, systolic bruit over the renal artery in the upper abdomen, reduced urine output, and an elevated renin level.

2 Renin stimulates formation of angiotensinogen in the liver. Angiotensinogen changes into angiotensin I and then, in the lungs, converts to angiotensin II.

Check for headache, nausea, anorexia, an elevated renin level, and hypertension.

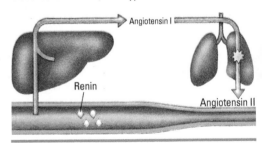

Angiotensin I

Renin

Angiotensin II

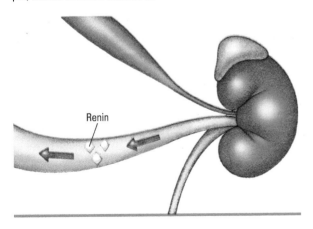

Renin

3 Angiotensin II is a potent vasoconstrictor and elevates blood pressure in the body.

Assess for hypertension, diminished urine output, albuminuria, hypokalemia, and hypernatremia.

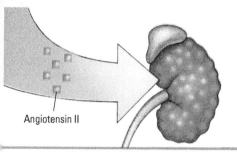

Angiotensin II

4 Angiotensin II stimulates the adrenal cortex to secrete aldosterone, which causes the nephrons to reabsorb sodium and water into the bloodstream, elevating blood volume and pressure further.

Expect worsening symptoms.

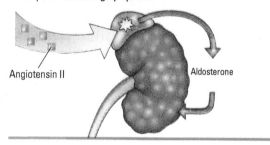

Angiotensin II   Aldosterone

5 Intermittent pressure diuresis causes excretion of sodium and water, reduced blood volume, and decreasing cardiac output.

Check for blood pressure that increases slowly, drops (but not as low as before), and then increases again. Headache, high urine specific gravity, hyponatremia, fatigue, and heart failure also occur.

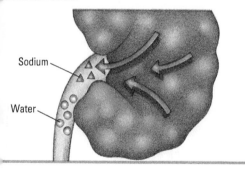

Sodium

Water

6 A high aldosterone level causes further sodium retention, but it can't curtail renin secretion. Excessive aldosterone and angiotensin II can damage renal tissue, leading to renal failure.

Expect to find hypertension, pitting edema, anemia, decreased level of consciousness, and elevated blood urea nitrogen and serum creatinine levels.

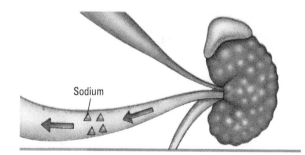

Sodium

What to look for

* Flank pain
* Systolic bruit over the renal artery in the abdomen
* Reduced urine output
* Headache
* Nausea
* Anorexia
* Anxiety
* Hypertension
* Altered level of consciousness
* Pitting edema

Lower urinary tract infection

A lower urinary tract infection (UTI), also called cystitis, is a localized bacterial infection in the bladder. The bladder and urethra become inflamed and edematous, causing specific types of symptoms. Females are more susceptible to UTI. One in five women reports having had a urinary tract infection sometime in her life.

"I'm hydrating....Lots of water flushes out the bacteria!"

How it happens

In UTI, bacteria invade the urinary tract. Most commonly, bacteria from the rectum enter the urethra and travel up to the bladder. The bacteria cause an inflammation reaction in the bladder, which results in swelling of the urethra. Females are more susceptible to UTI because of the anatomical proximity of the rectum and urethra. Bacteria easily invade the urethra and travel up into the bladder. Urine is a good medium for bacterial growth. The most common bacterium found in UTI is *E. coli*. Other bacteria include *Klebsiella pneumoniae*, *Proteus mirabilis*, *Enterococcus*, and *Staphylococcus saprophyticus*.

risky business

What to look for

- Dysuria (burning on urination)
- Frequency (needing to urinate frequently)
- Urgency (feeling of inability to hold urine)
- Suprapubic tenderness
- Foul-smelling urine
- White blood cells and red blood cells in urine

Risk Factors

- Sexual intercourse
- Use of a diaphragm or spermicide
- Poor perineal hygiene
- Tight undergarments
- Benign prostatic hyperplasia
- Pregnancy

- Kidney stone
- Urinary catheterization
- Pelvic examination
- Vesicourethral reflux (commo anatomic variation at the junction of the ureter and bladder)
- Kidney transplant

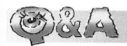

Able to label?

What classification of kidney injury occurs at each site?

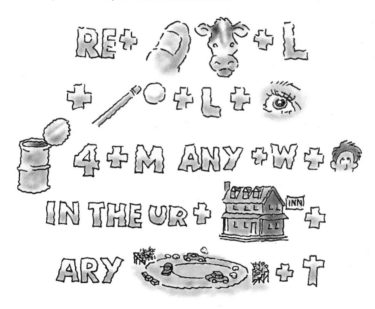

Lack of circulation to the
kidney is classified as (1)

Lack of urine outflow is
classified as (2)

Injury to kidney parenchyma
is classified as (3)

Riddle

Solve the riddle to discover the place where you'll find a renal disorder.

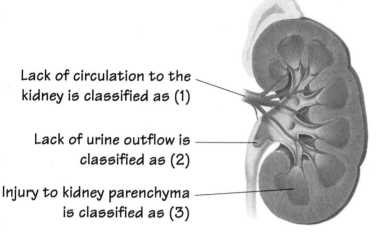

Riddle: Renal calculi can form anywhere in the urinary tract.

Answers: Able to label? 1. pre-renal dysfunction, 2. post-renal dysfunction, 3. intra-renal dysfunction.

Selected References

Colgan, R., & Williams, M. (2011). Diagnosis and treatment of acute uncomplicated cystitis. *American Family Physician, 84*(7), 771–776.

Colgan, R., Williams, M., & Johnson, J. R. (2011). Diagnosis and treatment of acute pyelonephritis in women. *American Family Physician, 84*(5), 519–526.

Grigoryan, L., Trautner, B. W., & Gupta, K. (2014). Diagnosis and management of urinary tract infections in the outpatient setting: A review. *Journal of the American Medical Association, 312*(16), 1677–1684.

Guirguis-Blake, J. (2014). Preventing recurrent nephrolithiasis in adults. *American Family Physician, 89*(6), 461–463.

Hinkle, J., & Cheever, K. (2014). *Brunner & Suddarth's textbook of medical surgical nursing* (13th ed.). Philadelphia, PA: Lippincott Williams & Wilkins.

Kumar, V., Abbas, A., & Aster, J. (2015). *Robbins & Cotran pathologic basis of disease* (9th ed.). Philadelphia, PA: Elsevier-Saunders.

National Institutes of Health. U.S. National Library of Medicine. Medline Plus. Glomerulonephritis. Retrieved from: http://www.nlm.nih.gov/medlineplus/ency/article/000484.htm on May 12, 2015.

National Kidney Foundation. (2015). Hydronephrosis. Retrieved from: https://www.kidney.org/atoz/content/hydronephrosis on May 20, 2015.

Rahman, M., Shad, F., & Smith, M. C. (2012). Acute kidney injury: A guide to diagnosis and management. *American Family Physician, 86*(7), 631–639.

Srivastava, A., & Patel, N. (2014). Autosomal dominant polycystic kidney disease. *American Family Physician, 90*(5), 303–307.

Chapter 11

Integumentary disorders

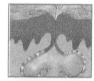
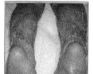
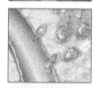

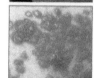

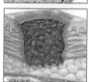
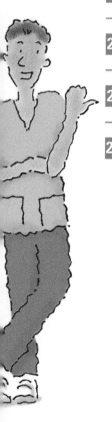

Acne

Integumentary

Acne is a chronic inflammatory disease of the sebaceous glands. It's usually associated with a high rate of sebum secretion and occurs on areas of the body that contain sebaceous glands, such as the face, neck, chest, back, and shoulders. There are two types of acne:

Inflammatory, in which the hair follicle is blocked by sebum, causing bacteria to grow and eventually rupture the follicle

Noninflammatory, in which the follicle doesn't rupture but remains dilated

How it happens

1
Excessive sebum production

Androgens stimulate sebaceous gland growth and the production of sebum, which is secreted into dilated hair follicles that contain bacteria.

2
Increased shedding of epithelial cells

The bacteria, usually *Propionibacterium acnes* and *Staphylococcus epidermidis,* are normal skin flora that secrete the enzyme lipase. This enzyme interacts with sebum to produce free fatty acids, which provoke inflammation.

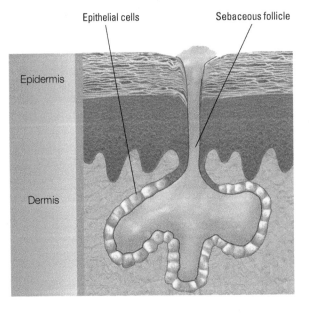

Epithelial cells   Sebaceous follicle

Epidermis

Dermis

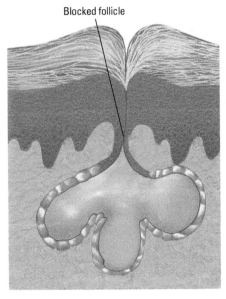

Blocked follicle

age-old story

Age and acne

Acne occurs in both males and females. Acne vulgaris develops in 80% to 90% of adolescents or young adults, primarily between ages 15 and 18.

Although lesions can appear as early as age 8, acne primarily affects adolescents. Sorry, guys!

Adolescent facial acne

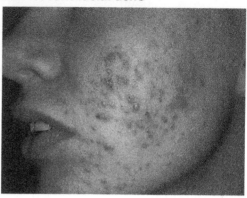

3

Inflammatory response in follicle

Hair follicles also produce more keratin, which joins with the sebum to form a plug in the dilated follicle.

Ruptured follicle

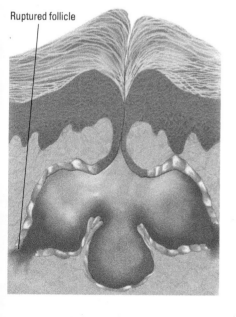

What to look for

The acne plug may appear as:
• A closed comedone, or whitehead (may be protruding from the follicle and covered by the epidermis)
• An open comedone, or blackhead (protruding from the follicle and not covered by the epidermis; melanin or pigment of the follicle causes the black color)
• Inflammation
• Acne pustules, papules, or, in severe forms, acne cysts or abscesses

Comedones of acne

Closed comedo (whitehead)

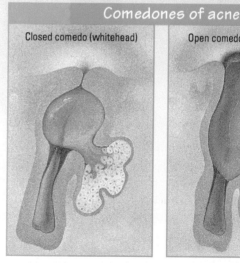

Open comedo (blackhead)

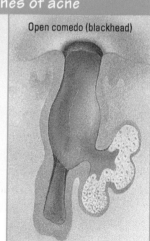

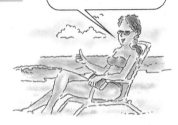

I'd better be careful, or I'll get a superficial partial-thickness burn…

Burns

Burns are classified as superficial partial thickness (first degree), deep partial thickness (second degree), full thickness (third degree), and full thickness involving muscle, bone, and interstitial tissue (fourth degree).

How it happens

The injuring agent denatures cellular proteins. Some cells die because of traumatic or ischemic necrosis. Loss of collagen cross-linking also occurs with denaturation, creating abnormal osmotic and hydrostatic pressure gradients, which cause the movement of intravascular fluid into interstitial spaces. Cellular injury triggers the release of mediators of inflammation, contributing to local and, in the case of major burns, systemic increases in capillary permeability. Specific pathophysiologic events depend on the burn's cause and classification.

Superficial partial-thickness burns

A superficial partial-thickness burn causes localized injury or destruction to the epidermis only by direct (such as chemical spill) or indirect (such as sunlight) contact. The barrier function of the skin remains intact.

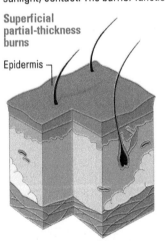

Superficial partial-thickness burns

Epidermis

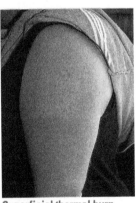

Superficial thermal burn (sunburn)

Deep partial-thickness burns

Deep partial-thickness burns involve destruction to the epidermis and some dermis. Thin-walled, fluid-filled blisters develop within a few minutes of the injury along with mild to

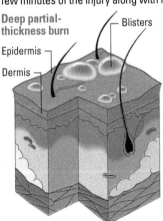

Deep partial-thickness burn

Blisters

Epidermis

Dermis

What to look for

Superficial partial-thickness burn
* Localized pain and erythema, usually without blisters in the first 24 hours, caused by injury from direct or indirect contact with a burn source
* Chills, headache, localized edema, and nausea and vomiting (with more severe superficial partial-thickness burn)
* Thin-walled, fluid-filled blisters appearing within minutes of the injury, with mild to moderate edema and pain (with deep partial-thickness burn)
* White, waxy appearance to damaged area (deep partial-thickness burn)

> Is it black or white or in-between? Color can be a major assessment factor when it comes to burns. A white waxy burn is a superficial partial-thickness burn. A leathery black or silver-colored burn is full thickness.

Age and burns

Burn victims younger than age 4 and older than age 60 experience a higher incidence of complications and thus a higher mortality rate.

moderate edema and pain. As these blisters break, the nerve endings become exposed to the air. Pain and tactile responses remain intact, so subsequent treatments are painful. The barrier function of the skin is lost.

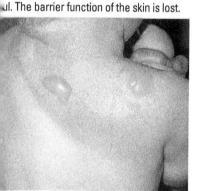

Deep partial-thickness burn (sunburn)

Full-thickness burns

A major full-thickness burn affects every body system and organ. A full-thickness burn extends through the epidermis and dermis and into the subcutaneous tissue layer. If the burn is fourth degree, muscle, bone, and interstitial tissues would also be involved. Within hours, fluids and protein shift from capillary to interstitial spaces, causing edema. The immediate immunologic response to the burn injury makes burn wound sepsis a potential threat. Lastly, an increase in calorie demand after the burn injury increases metabolic rate.

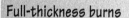
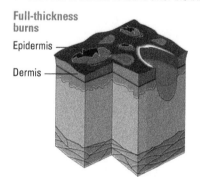

Full-thickness burns

Epidermis

Dermis

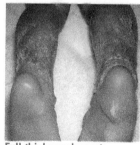

Full-thickness burns to the legs

Full-thickness burn

White, brown, or black leathery tissue and visible thrombosed vessels due to destruction of skin elasticity (the dorsum of the hand is the most common site of thrombosed veins), without blisters

Silver-colored, raised area, usually at the site of electrical contact (with electrical burn)

Singed nasal hairs, mucosal burns, voice changes, coughing, wheezing, soot in mouth or nose, and darkened sputum with smoke inhalation and pulmonary damage).

Cellulitis

Cellulitis is an infection of the dermis or subcutaneous layer of the skin. It may follow damage to the skin, such as a bite or wound. As the cellulitis spreads, fever, erythema, and lymphangitis may occur.

If cellulitis is treated in a timely manner, the prognosis is usually good.

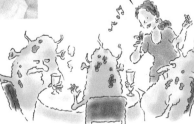

age-old story

Age and cellulitis

Cellulitis of the lower extremity is more likely to develop into thrombophlebitis in an elderly patient.

How it happens

As the offending organism invades the compromised area, it overwhelms the defensive cells (neutrophils, eosinophils, basophils, and mast cells) that break down the cellular components, which normally contain and localize the inflammation. As cellulitis progresses, the organism invades tissue around the initial wound site.

Phases of acute inflammatory response

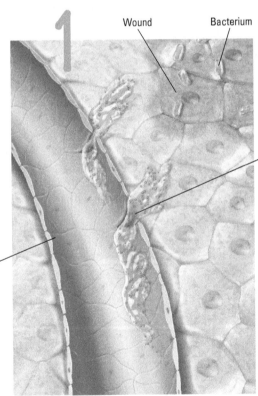

Wound

Bacterium

Increased blood flow carrying plasma proteins and fluid to the injured tissue

Blood vessel

I've got you under my skin— and I want you out!

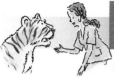

Risk factors for cellulitis

- Diabetes
- Immunodeficiency
- Impaired circulation
- Neuropathy

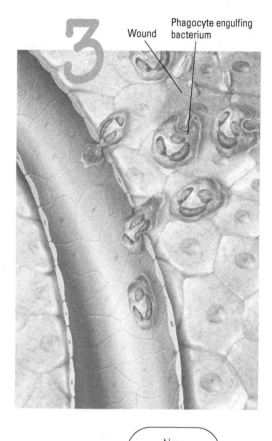

Wound

Phagocyte engulfing bacterium

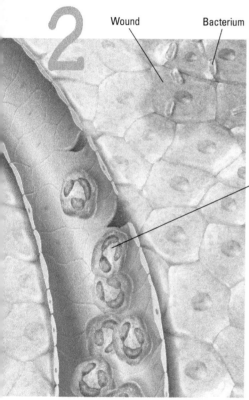

Wound

Bacterium

Movement of defensive white blood cells to injured tissue

Recognizing cellulitis

The classic signs of cellulitis are erythema and edema surrounding the initial wound. The tissue is warm to the touch.

Initial wound

Surrounding erythema and edema

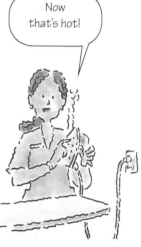

Now that's hot!

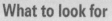

Contact dermatitis

Contact dermatitis commonly appears as a sharply demarcated inflammation of the skin resulting from contact with an irritating chemical or atopic allergen (a substance producing an allergic reaction in the skin). It can also appear as an irritation of the skin resulting from contact with concentrated substances to which the skin is sensitive, such as perfumes, soaps, chemicals, or metals and alloys (for instance, the nickel used in jewelry).

How it happens

1

Antigen contacts skin.

2

Antigen is processed by antigen-presenting cell called Langerhans cell.

Langerhans' cell

3

Processed antigen presented to the T cells. Processing, presentation, and sensitization takes 24 hours.

Hapten-carrier complex

T c

Sensitized T cells

4

Sensitized T cells enter a lymphatic vessel.

Lymphatic vessel

5

Sensitized T cells transported to regional lymph nodes, where T-cell hyperplasia is induced.

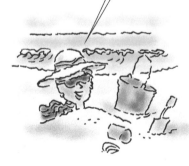

Your patients don't have to hide their dermatitis from the world! They just have to be careful of their sensitive skin!

What to look for

- Erythema and small vesicles that ooze, scale, and itch (due to mild irritants and allergens)
- Blisters and ulcerations (due to strong irritants)
- Clearly defined lesions, with straight lines following points of contact (classic allergic response)
- Marked erythema, blistering, and edema of affected areas (severe allergic reaction)

Contact dermatitis from nickel of watch on skin

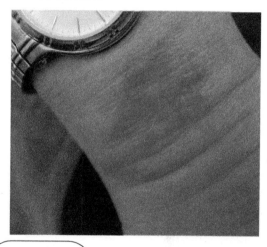

6

Sensitized T cells return to dermis and epidermis.

Lymph node

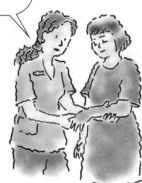

Looks like you've been scratching again!

Herpes zoster

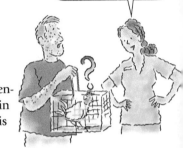

I said, "It looks like you have chickenpox," not "a chicken in a box."

Herpes zoster, also called *shingles*, is an acute inflammation caused by infection with human herpesvirus 3 (varicella-zoster virus [VZV], or chickenpox virus). It usually occurs in adults and produces localized vesicular skin lesions and severe neuralgic pain in peripheral areas. Complete recovery is common, but scarring may occur as well as vision impairment (with corneal damage) or persistent neuralgia.

How it happens

An individual (usually a child) develops chickenpox through droplet transmission or inhalation of the varicella or chickenpox virus. The virus initially causes a "silent" infection of the nasopharynx. This infection progresses to viremia, seeding of fixed macrophages, and dissemination of VZV to the skin (the rash seen in chickenpox).

After the initial infection, the virus lays dormant in the dorsal spinal ganglion, where it remains for many years. The virus is reactivated, probably because of decreased cellular immunity, and spreads from ganglia along the sensory nerves to the peripheral nerves of sensory dermatomes, causing shingles.

1
Varicella-zoster virus (chickenpox)

2
Non-immune individual (usually a child)

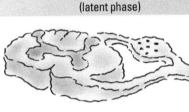

3
Virus in dorsal spinal ganglion (latent phase)

Dormant?! I can't believe there's *anything* dormant in this little guy.

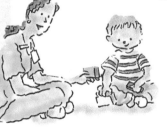

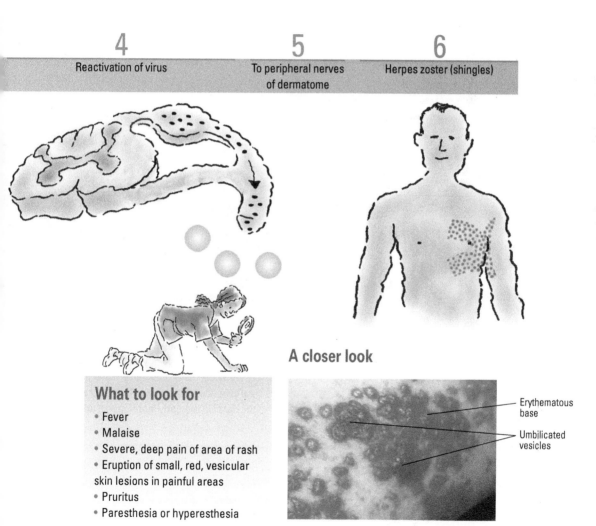

4
Reactivation of virus

5
To peripheral nerves
of dermatome

6
Herpes zoster (shingles)

What to look for

- Fever
- Malaise
- Severe, deep pain of area of rash
- Eruption of small, red, vesicular
skin lesions in painful areas
- Pruritus
- Paresthesia or hyperesthesia

A closer look

Erythematous
base

Umbilicated
vesicles

Malignant melanoma

Malignant melanoma is the most lethal skin cancer. It accounts for 1% to 2% of all malignant tumors, and it's slightly more common in women than men.

How it happens

Malignant melanoma arises from melanocytes (cells that synthesize the pigment melanin). In addition to the skin, melanocytes are also found in the meninges, alimentary canal, respiratory tract, and lymph nodes.

Melanoma spreads through the lymphatic and vascular systems and metastasizes to the regional lymph nodes, skin, liver, lungs, and central nervous system. In most patients, superficial lesions are curable, but deeper lesions are more likely to metastasize.

Up to 70% of malignant melanomas arise from a preexisting nevus, sometimes called a "beauty mark" or mole.

Understanding skin cancer

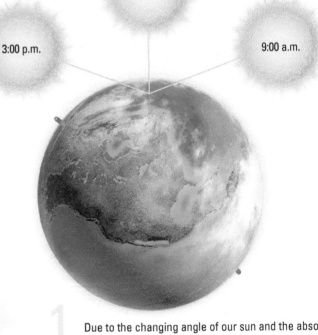

Noon

3:00 p.m.

9:00 a.m.

Due to the changing angle of our sun and the absorption of solar radiation by our atmosphere, the intensity of ultraviolet (UV) radiation striking the surface of the earth at noon is twice as strong as radiation striking the earth in the early morning and late afternoon.

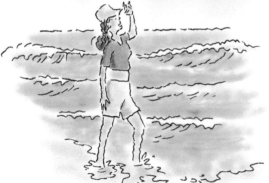

Age and malignant melanoma

Malignant melanoma is unusual in children, and occurs most commonly between ages 40 and 50. However, the incidence in younger age-groups is increasing because of increased sun exposure or, possibly, a decrease in the ozone layer.

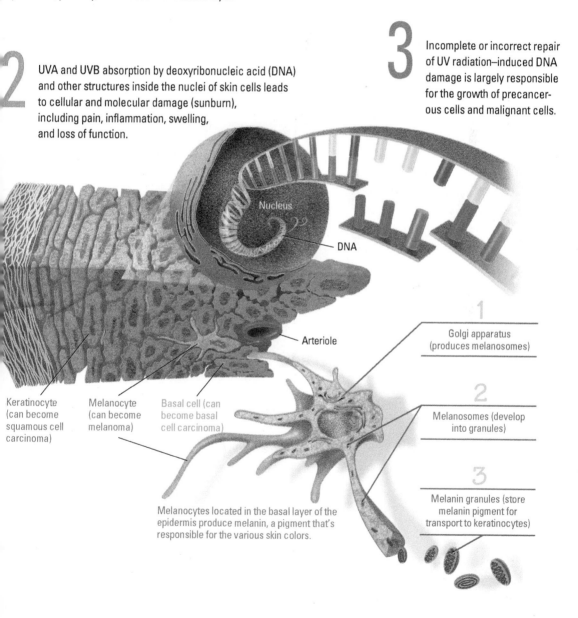

2 UVA and UVB absorption by deoxyribonucleic acid (DNA) and other structures inside the nuclei of skin cells leads to cellular and molecular damage (sunburn), including pain, inflammation, swelling, and loss of function.

3 Incomplete or incorrect repair of UV radiation–induced DNA damage is largely responsible for the growth of precancerous cells and malignant cells.

Nucleus

DNA

Arteriole

Keratinocyte (can become squamous cell carcinoma)

Melanocyte (can become melanoma)

Basal cell (can become basal cell carcinoma)

Melanocytes located in the basal layer of the epidermis produce melanin, a pigment that's responsible for the various skin colors.

1 Golgi apparatus (produces melanosomes)

2 Melanosomes (develop into granules)

3 Melanin granules (store melanin pigment for transport to keratinocytes)

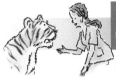

risky business

Risk factors for melanoma

- Excessive exposure to sunlight
- Increased size of nevus
- Tendency to freckle from the sun
- Hormonal factors such as pregnancy

- A family history or past history of melanoma
- Red hair, fair skin, blue eyes, susceptibility to sunburn, and Celtic or Scandinavian ancestry (Melanoma is rare in blacks.)

> Did you say red hair, fair skin, and blue eyes? Drats! Bring me the sunscreen!

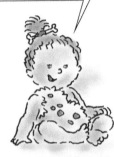

What to look for

Changes to a preexisting skin lesion or nevus
- Enlarges
- Changes color
- Becomes inflamed or sore
- Itches
- Ulcerates
- Bleeds
- Changes texture
- Shows signs of surrounding pigment regression

A closer look

Malignant melanoma can arise on normal skin or from an existing mole. If not treated promptly, it can spread to other areas of skin, lymph nodes, or internal organs.

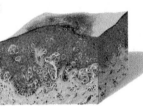

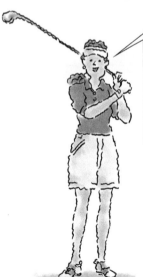

> Common sites for malignant melanoma are the head and neck in men and the legs in women. So, wear that sunblock or put on a hat and pants!

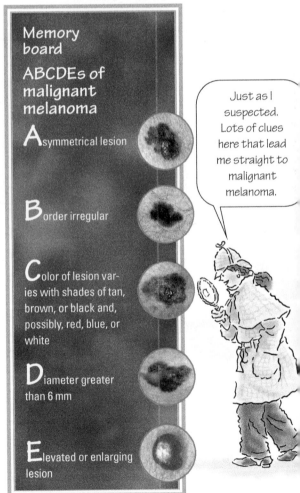

Memory board

ABCDEs of malignant melanoma

Asymmetrical lesion

Border irregular

Color of lesion varies with shades of tan, brown, or black and, possibly, red, blue, or white

Diameter greater than 6 mm

Elevated or enlarging lesion

> Just as I suspected. Lots of clues here that lead me straight to malignant melanoma.

Pressure ulcers

Pressure ulcers, commonly called pressure sores or bedsores, are localized areas of cellular necrosis that occur most often in the skin and subcutaneous tissue over bony prominences. These ulcers may be superficial (caused by local skin irritation with subsequent surface maceration) or deep (originating in underlying tissue). Deep lesions commonly remain undetected until they penetrate the skin, but by then, they have usually caused subcutaneous damage.

Most pressure ulcers develop over five body locations:

1 Sacral area   **2** Lateral malleolus   **3** Ischial tuberosity   **4** Greater trochanter   **5** Heel

Collectively, these areas account for 95% of all pressure ulcer sites. Patients who have contractures are at an increased risk for developing pressure ulcers because of the added pressure on the tissue and the alignment of the bones.

Pressure ulcers are categorized as suspected deep tissue injury, stage I, stage II, stage III, stage IV, or unstageable.

How it happens

A pressure ulcer is caused by an injury to the skin and its underlying tissues. The pressure exerted on the area causes ischemia and hypoxemia to the affected tissues because of decreased blood flow to the site.

As the capillaries collapse, thrombosis occurs, which subsequently leads to tissue edema and then tissue necrosis.

Ischemia also adds to an accumulation of waste products at the site, which in turn leads to the production of toxins. The toxins further break down the tissue and eventually lead to the death of the cells.

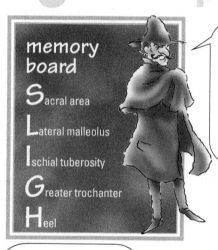

memory board

Sacral area
Lateral malleolus
Ischial tuberosity
Greater trochanter
Heel

Here's a SLIGH way to remember the five body locations where pressure ulcers commonly develop.

When ischemia is in town, there's always an accumulation of waste products.

age-old story

Age and pressure ulcers

Age plays a role in the incidence of pressure ulcers. Muscle is lost with aging, and skin elasticity decreases. Both of these factors increase the risk of developing pressure ulcers.

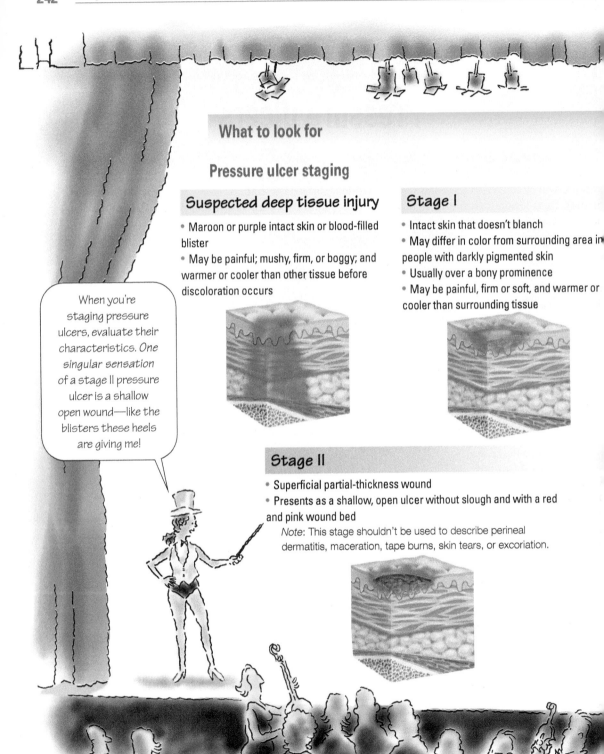

What to look for

Pressure ulcer staging

Suspected deep tissue injury

- Maroon or purple intact skin or blood-filled blister
- May be painful; mushy, firm, or boggy; and warmer or cooler than other tissue before discoloration occurs

Stage I

- Intact skin that doesn't blanch
- May differ in color from surrounding area in people with darkly pigmented skin
- Usually over a bony prominence
- May be painful, firm or soft, and warmer or cooler than surrounding tissue

Stage II

- Superficial partial-thickness wound
- Presents as a shallow, open ulcer without slough and with a red and pink wound bed

  Note: This stage shouldn't be used to describe perineal dermatitis, maceration, tape burns, skin tears, or excoriation.

When you're staging pressure ulcers, evaluate their characteristics. One singular sensation of a stage II pressure ulcer is a shallow open wound—like the blisters these heels are giving me!

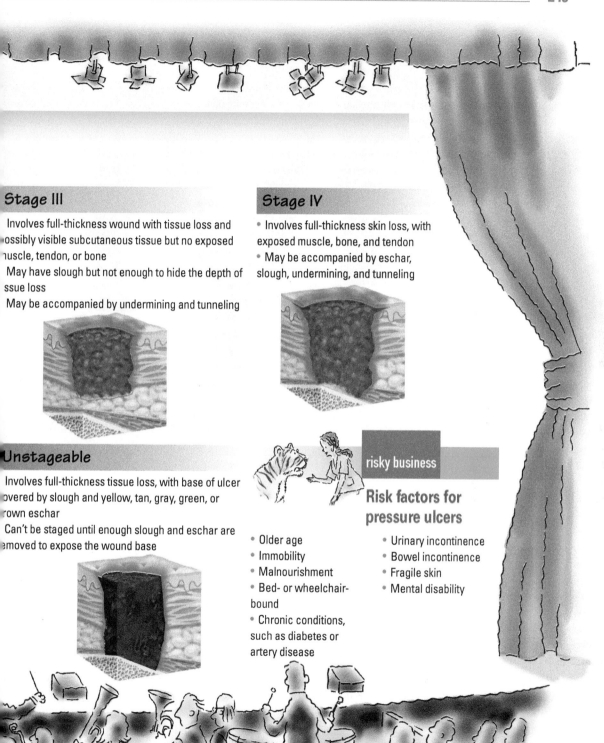

Stage III

Involves full-thickness wound with tissue loss and possibly visible subcutaneous tissue but no exposed muscle, tendon, or bone

May have slough but not enough to hide the depth of tissue loss

May be accompanied by undermining and tunneling

Stage IV

- Involves full-thickness skin loss, with exposed muscle, bone, and tendon
- May be accompanied by eschar, slough, undermining, and tunneling

Unstageable

Involves full-thickness tissue loss, with base of ulcer covered by slough and yellow, tan, gray, green, or brown eschar

Can't be staged until enough slough and eschar are removed to expose the wound base

risky business

Risk factors for pressure ulcers

- Older age
- Immobility
- Malnourishment
- Bed- or wheelchair-bound
- Chronic conditions, such as diabetes or artery disease

- Urinary incontinence
- Bowel incontinence
- Fragile skin
- Mental disability

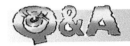

Show and tell

Identify the three types of burns in each illustration and indicate their characteristics.

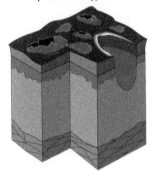
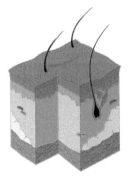
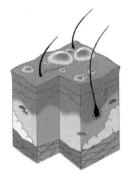

1. _____

_____

_____

_____

_____

_____

_____

2. _____

_____

_____

_____

_____

_____

_____

3. _____

_____

_____

_____

_____

_____

Matchmaker

Match the definitions with their corresponding disorders.

1. Most lethal skin cancer _____

2. Localized areas of cellular necrosis that are most common over bony prominences _____

3. Chronic inflammatory disease of the sebaceous glands _____

4. Inflammation or irritation of the skin due to contact with irritating chemical or atopic allergen _____

5. Infection of the dermis or subcutaneous layer of the skin _____

6. Acute inflammation caused by infection with herpesvirus _____

A. Cellulitis

B. Herpes zoster

C. Acne

D. Contact dermatitis

E. Malignant melanoma

F. Pressure ulcers

Answers: **Show and tell 1.** Full-thickness; extends through the epidermis and dermis and into the subcutaneous tissue layer **2.** superficial partial-thickness; causes localized injury or destruction to the epidermis only **3.** deep partial-thickness; involves destruction to the epidermis and some dermis

Matchmaker 1. E, **2.** F, **3.** C, **4.** D, **5.** A, **6.** B

Selected References

Bluestein, D., & Javaheri, A. (2008). Pressure ulcers: Prevention, evaluation, and management. *American Family Physician, 78*(10), 1186–1194.

Calianno, C., & O'Shea, S. (2013). Herpes zoster in older adults. *Nurse Practitioner, 38*(8), 10–14.

Fashner, J., & Bell, A. L. (2011). Herpes zoster and postherpetic neuralgia: Prevention and management. *American Family Physician, 83*(12), 1432–1437.

Fogel, A. L., Longmire, M., Rieger, K. E., & Sarin, K. Y. (2015). A subdermal source: Contact dermatitis. *American Journal of Medicine, 128*(6), 578–581.

Gould, D. (2014). Varicella zoster virus: Chickenpox and shingles. *Nursing Standard, 28*(33), 52–58.

Gunderson, C. G. (2011). Cellulitis: Definition, etiology, and clinical features. *American Journal of Medicine, 124*(12), 1113–1122.

Ibrahimi, O. A., Sakamoto, G. K., & Lee, J. J. (2010). Acute onset vesicular rash. Herpes zoster. *American Family Physician, 82*(7), 815–816.

Kocher, J. (2013). Prevention of herpes zoster in older adults. *American Family Physician, 88*(9), 578.

Kundu, R. V., & Patterson, S. (2013). Dermatologic conditions in skin of color: Part I. Special considerations for common skin disorders. *American Family Physician, 87*(12), 850–856.

Lloyd, E. C., Rodgers, B. C., Michener, M., & Williams, M. S. (2012). Outpatient burns: Prevention and care. *American Family Physician, 85*(1), 25–32.

Perkins, A., & Duffy, R. L. (2015). Atypical moles: Diagnosis and management. *American Family Physician, 91*(11), 762–767.

Rowan, M. P., Cancio, L. C., Elster, E. A., Burmeister, D. M., Rose, L. F., Natesan, S., …, Chung, K. K. (2015). Burn wound healing and treatment: Review and advancements. *Critical Care, 19*(1), 243–260.

Rubin, K. M. (2013). Management of primary cutaneous and metastatic melanoma. *Seminars in Oncology Nursing, 29*(3), 195–205.

Shenenberger, D. W. (2012). Cutaneous malignant melanoma: A primary care perspective. *American Family Physician, 85*(2), 161–168.

Titus, S., & Hodge, J. (2012). Diagnosis and treatment of acne. *American Family Physician, 86*(8), 734–740.

Usatine, R. P., & Riojas, M. (2010). Diagnosis and management of contact dermatitis. *American Family Physician, 82*(3), 249–255.

Wilson, D. D. (2014). Herpes zoster (shingles). *Nurse Practitioner, 39*(5), 15–16.

Chapter 12

Reproductive disorders

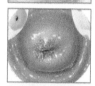
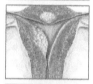

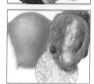
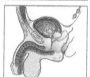
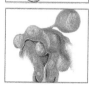

Benign prostatic hyperplasia

Reproductive

Although most men age 50 and older have some prostatic enlargement, in benign prostatic hyperplasia (BPH)—also known as *benign prostatic hypertrophy*—the prostate gland enlarges enough to compress the urethra and cause overt urinary obstruction.

How it happens

Regardless of the cause, BPH begins with nonmalignant changes in periurethral glandular tissue. The growth of the fibroadenomatous nodules (masses of fibrous glandular tissue) progresses to compress the remaining normal gland (nodular hyperplasia). The hyperplastic tissue is mostly glandular, with some fibrous stroma and smooth muscle.

As the prostate enlarges, it obstructs urinary outflow by compressing the prostatic urethra. Periodic increases in sympathetic stimulation of the smooth muscle of the prostatic urethra and bladder neck also occur. Progressive bladder distention occurs due to retained urine. This retained urine may lead to calculus formation or cystitis.

Prostatic enlargement

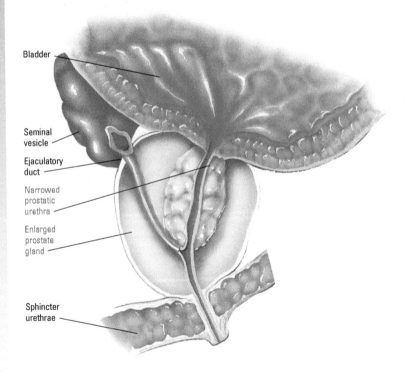

Bladder

Seminal vesicle

Ejaculatory duct

Narrowed prostatic urethra

Enlarged prostate gland

Sphincter urethrae

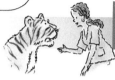

age-old story

Age and BPH

BPH is common, affecting up to 50% of men over age 50 and 80% of men over age 80.

> I said, "Have you had your prostate checked lately?"

risky business

Risk factors for BPH

- Age
- Family history of BPH

Nodular hyperplasia of the prostate

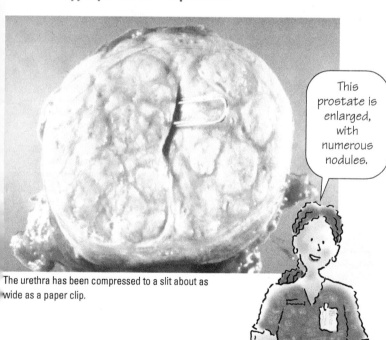

> This prostate is enlarged, with numerous nodules.

The urethra has been compressed to a slit about as wide as a paper clip.

What to look for

Signs and symptoms of BPH depend on the extent of prostatic enlargement and the lobes affected. Characteristically, the condition starts with a group of symptoms known as *prostatism*, which are caused by enlargement and include

- Reduced urine stream caliber and force
- Urinary hesitancy
- Difficulty starting micturition (resulting in straining, feeling of incomplete voiding, and an interrupted stream)

As the obstruction increases, it causes:

- Frequent urination with nocturia
- Sense of urgency
- Dribbling of urine
- Urine retention
- Urinary incontinence
- Possible hematuria
- Possible urinary tract infection
- Enlarged prostate palpable on digital rectal exam by clinician

Breast cancer

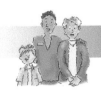

age-old story

Age and breast cancer

Although the disease may develop any time after puberty, 70% of cases occur in women older than age 50.

Breast cancer is the most common cancer in women. Breast cancer ranks second among cancer deaths in women, behind cancer of the lung.

How it happens

Slow-growing breast cancer spreads by way of the lymphatic system and the bloodstream, eventually to the other breast, the chest wall, liver, bone, and brain.

Most breast cancers arise from the ductal epithelium. Tumors of the infiltrating ductal type don't enlarge dramatically but metastasize early.

> Breast cancer occurs more frequently in the left breast than the right and more commonly in the outer upper quadrant.

Types of breast cancer

Ductal carcinoma in situ

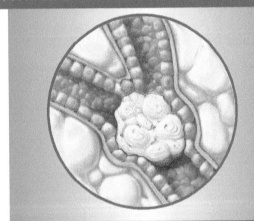

Infiltrating (invasive) ductal carcinoma

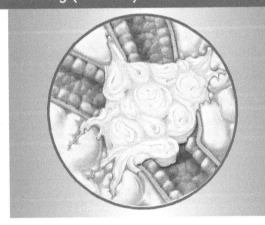

Classifying breast cancer

Breast cancer is classified by histologic appearance and location of the lesion:
- Adenocarcinoma—arises from the glandular epithelium
- Intraductal—occurs within the ducts (including Paget disease of the breast)
- Infiltrating—appears in parenchymal tissue of the breast
- Inflammatory (rare)—overlying skin becomes edematous, inflamed, and indurated; reflects rapid tumor growth
- Lobular carcinoma in situ—involves glandular lobes
- Medullary or circumscribed—appears as a large tumor, with rapid growth rate

Staging of breast cancer

Stage I

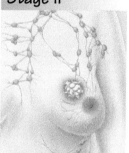

Stage II

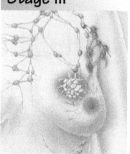

Stage III

Stage IV

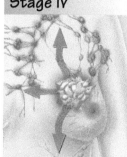

In stage I, the tumor is less than 2 cm in size; there are no axillary or other metastases.

In stage II, the tumor is greater than 2 cm in size; there may be metastasis to the axillary lymph nodes, but it doesn't extend into other areas.

In stage III, the tumor is greater than 5 cm in size; there is metastasis to axillary lymph nodes but no other metastasis.

In stage IV, the tumor can be any size, supraclavicular or infraclavicular lymph nodes are affected, and there's distant metastasis.

risky business

Risk factors for breast cancer

Higher risk
* Family history of breast cancer, particularly first-degree relatives (mother or sister)
* Genetic mutations in BRCA1 and BRCA2 genes (suggest genetic predisposition)
* Long menses (menses beginning early or menopause beginning late)
* No history of pregnancy
* History of breast cancer
* History of endometrial or ovarian cancer

* Exposure to low-level ionizing radiation
* Alcohol use
* Extended use of hormone replacement therapy
* Obesity
* Smoking

Lower risk
* History of pregnancy before age 20
* History of multiple pregnancies
* History of breast-feeding
* Native American or Asian ethnicity

> Genetic mutations are just one of the major risk factors for breast cancer. OK, everyone, let's see what we end up with when everyone does left foot blue.

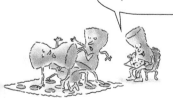

Carcinoma of the breast

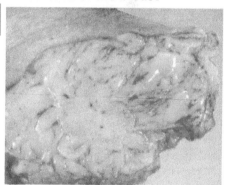

What to look for

* Thickening of the breast tissue
* Painless lump or mass in the breast
* Nipple retraction
* Hard, nodular, immobile mass
* Scaly skin around the nipple
* Skin changes; dimpling of skin or a skin change called peau d'orange common
* Erythema
* Clear, milky, or bloody discharge
* Edema in the arm, indicating advanced nodal involvement
* Cervical supraclavicular and axillary node enlargement
* Pain in the nipple or other areas of the breast
* Prominent superficial veins of breast

Cervical cancer

Cervical cancer is the third most common cancer of the female reproductive system and is classified as either invasive or microinvasive. Preinvasive disease, also known as *precancerous dysplasia, cervical intraepithelial carcinoma,* or *cervical cancer in situ,* is more frequent than invasive cancer and occurs more commonly in younger women.

How it happens

Preinvasive disease can range from mild cervical dysplasia (in which the lower third of the epithelium contains abnormal cells) to carcinoma in situ (in which the full thickness of epithelium contains abnormally proliferating cells).

In invasive carcinoma, cancer cells penetrate the basement membrane and can spread directly to adjacent pelvic structures or disseminate to distant sites by lymphatic routes.

A closer look

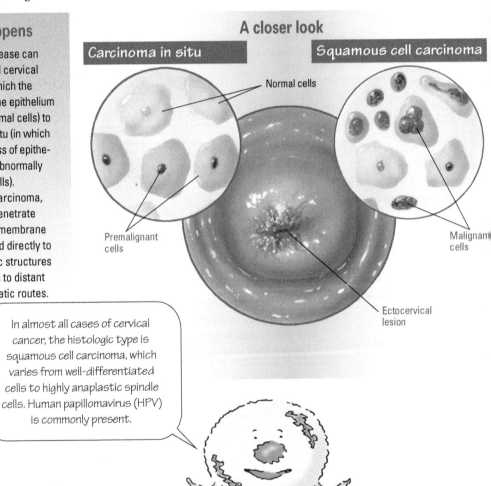

Carcinoma in situ

Squamous cell carcinoma

Normal cells

Premalignant cells

Malignant cells

Ectocervical lesion

In almost all cases of cervical cancer, the histologic type is squamous cell carcinoma, which varies from well-differentiated cells to highly anaplastic spindle cells. Human papillomavirus (HPV) is commonly present.

Age and cervical cancer

Usually, invasive carcinoma occurs in women between ages 30 and 50; it rarely occurs in those younger than age 20.

What to look for

Preinvasive disease	Early invasive disease	Advanced disease
• Commonly no symptoms	• Abnormal or persistent vaginal bleeding • Postcoital pain and bleeding	• Pelvic pain • Vaginal leakage of urine and stool from a fistula • Anorexia, weight loss, and anemia

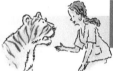

Risk factors for cervical cancer

• Frequent intercourse at a young age (younger than age 16)
• Multiple sexual partners
• Sexually transmitted infections (particularly human papillomavirus [HPV])
• Smoking
• Previous history of cervical dysplasia

Squamous cell carcinoma in the cervix

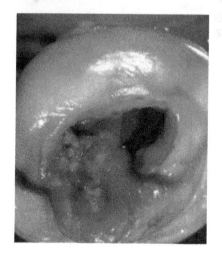

Endometrial cancer

Also known as *uterine cancer*, endometrial cancer is the most common gynecologic cancer.

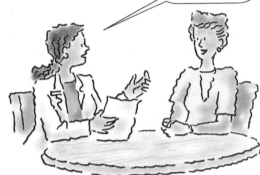

Endometrial cancer originates in the endometrium, which is the lining of the uterus.

How it happens

In most cases, endometrial cancer is an adenocarcinoma that metastasizes late, usually from the endometrium to the cervix, ovaries, fallopian tubes, and other peritoneal structures. It may spread to distant organs, such as the lungs and the brain, through the blood or lymphatic system. Lymph node involvement can also occur.

Progression of endometrial cancer

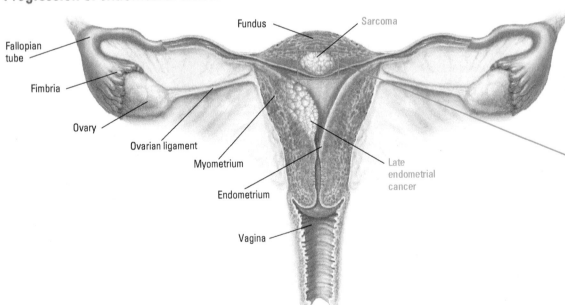

Fallopian tube

Fimbria

Ovary

Ovarian ligament

Myometrium

Endometrium

Vagina

Fundus

Sarcoma

Late endometrial cancer

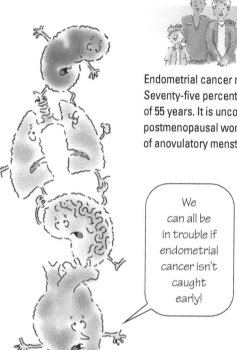

Age and endometrial cancer

Endometrial cancer most commonly affects postmenopausal women. Seventy-five percent of cases are diagnosed in women over the age of 55 years. It is uncommon in women under the age of 45 years. Most postmenopausal women who develop uterine cancer have a history of anovulatory menstrual cycles or other hormonal imbalance.

We can all be in trouble if endometrial cancer isn't caught early!

What to look for

- Uterine enlargement
- Persistent and unusual premenopausal bleeding
- Postmenopausal bleeding
- Pain and weight loss (advanced cancer)

Adenocarcinoma of the endometrium

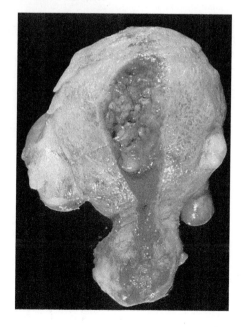

Advanced endometrial cancer

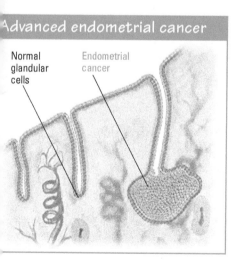

Normal glandular cells

Endometrial cancer

Endometriosis

Endometriosis is the presence of endometrial tissue outside the lining of the uterine cavity. Ectopic endometrial tissue is generally confined to the pelvic area, usually around the ovaries, uterovesical peritoneum, uterosacral ligaments, and the cul-de-sac, but it can appear anywhere in the body.

How it happens

The ectopic endometrial tissue responds to normal stimulation in the same way as does the endometrium, but more unpredictably. The endometrial cells respond to estrogen and progesterone with proliferation and secretion. During menstruation, the ectopic tissue bleeds, which causes inflammation of the surrounding tissue. This inflammation causes fibrosis, leading to adhesions that produce pain and infertility.

Pelvic endometriosis

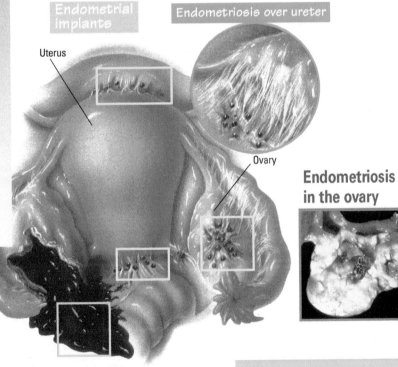

Endometrial implants

Endometriosis over ureter

Uterus

Ovary

Endometriosis in the ovary

Ruptured endometrial cyst of right ovary

What to look for

- Dysmenorrhea
- Abnormal uterine bleeding
- Infertility
- Pain that begins 5 to 7 days before menses peaks and lasts for 2 to 3 days

Common sites of endometriosis, with corresponding signs and symptoms

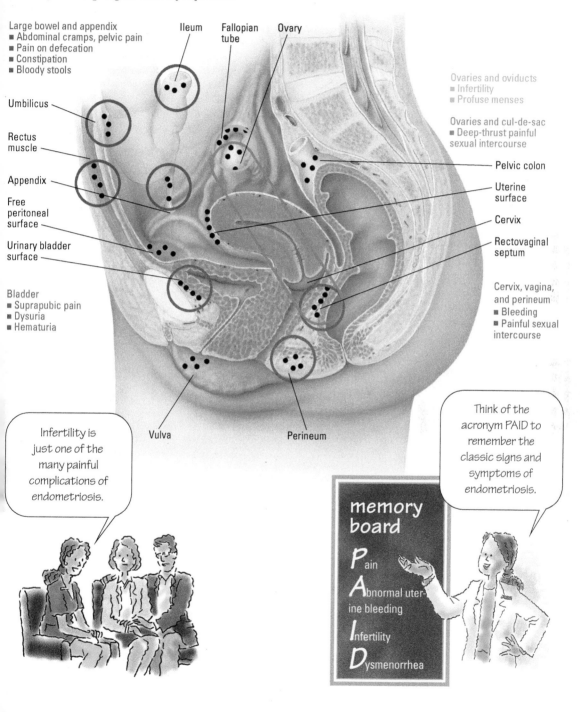

Large bowel and appendix
- Abdominal cramps, pelvic pain
- Pain on defecation
- Constipation
- Bloody stools

Ileum

Fallopian tube

Ovary

Umbilicus

Rectus muscle

Appendix

Free peritoneal surface

Urinary bladder surface

Bladder
- Suprapubic pain
- Dysuria
- Hematuria

Ovaries and oviducts
- Infertility
- Profuse menses

Ovaries and cul-de-sac
- Deep-thrust painful sexual intercourse

Pelvic colon

Uterine surface

Cervix

Rectovaginal septum

Cervix, vagina, and perineum
- Bleeding
- Painful sexual intercourse

Vulva

Perineum

Infertility is just one of the many painful complications of endometriosis.

Think of the acronym PAID to remember the classic signs and symptoms of endometriosis.

memory board

*P*ain

*A*bnormal uterine bleeding

*I*nfertility

*D*ysmenorrhea

Ovarian cancer

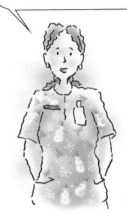

The prognosis for ovarian cancer is usually poor because ovarian tumors are difficult to diagnose and progress rapidly.

After cancers of the lung, breast, and colon, primary ovarian cancer ranks as the most common cause of cancer death among women in the United States. In women with previously treated breast cancer, metastatic ovarian cancer is more common than cancer of any other organ. The prognosis varies with the histologic type and staging of the disease.

How it happens

In ovarian cancer, primary epithelial tumors arise in the müllerian epithelium; germ cell tumors arise in the ovum; and sex cord tumors arise in the ovarian stroma. Ovarian tumors spread rapidly intraperitoneally by local extension or surface seeding and, occasionally, through the lymphatic system and the bloodstream. In most cases, extraperitoneal spread is through the diaphragm into the chest cavity, which may cause pleural effusions. Other metastasis is rare.

A closer look

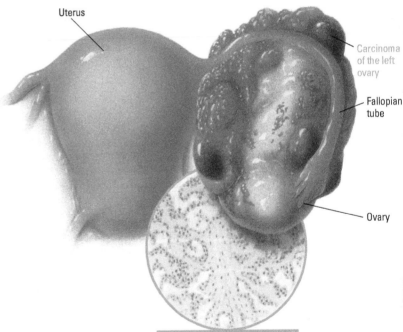

Uterus

Carcinoma of the left ovary

Fallopian tube

Ovary

Microscopic view of ovarian cancer cells

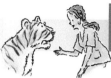

risky business

Risk factors for ovarian cancer

* Family history of ovarian cancer in close relatives
* Advancing age
* Obesity
* Use of Clomid for a period of time exceeding 1 year
* First full-term pregnancy after age 35
* History of breast cancer

* History of uterine or cervical cancer
* History of colorectal cancer
* Infertility
* Late menopause
* Long-term estrogen replacement therapy
* Starting menses at a young age (before age 12)
* BRCA1 or BRCA2 genetic mutation

What to look for

* Vague abdominal discomfort
* Urinary frequency
* Constipation
* Pain
* Feminizing or masculinizing effects
* Ascites
* Pleural effusions

Common metastatic sites for ovarian cancer

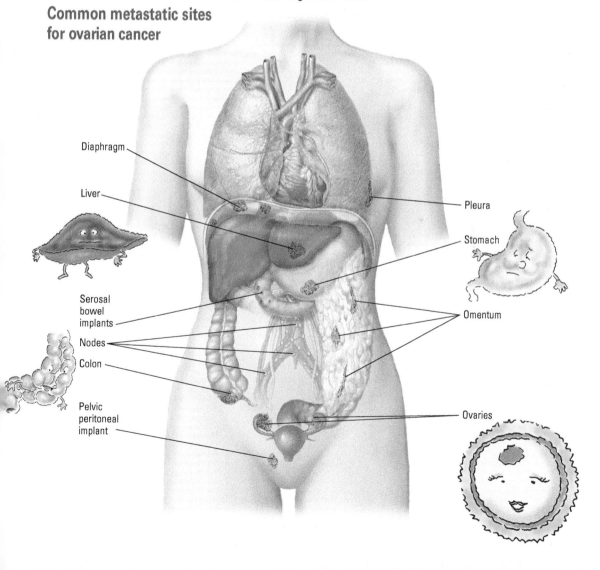

Diaphragm

Liver

Serosal bowel implants

Nodes

Colon

Pelvic peritoneal implant

Pleura

Stomach

Omentum

Ovaries

Ovarian cysts

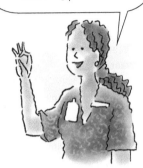

While ovarian cysts can be this small, they can cause big problems.

Ovarian cysts are usually nonneoplastic areas on an ovary that contain fluid or semisolid material. Commonly, ovarian cysts develop in areas where an egg comes to the surface of the ovary during germination and leaves behind a sac—these are called follicular or corpus luteal cysts. Although these cysts are usually small and produce no symptoms, they may require thorough investigation as possible sites of malignant change. Cysts may be single or multiple. The prognosis for nonneoplastic ovarian cysts is excellent.

How it happens

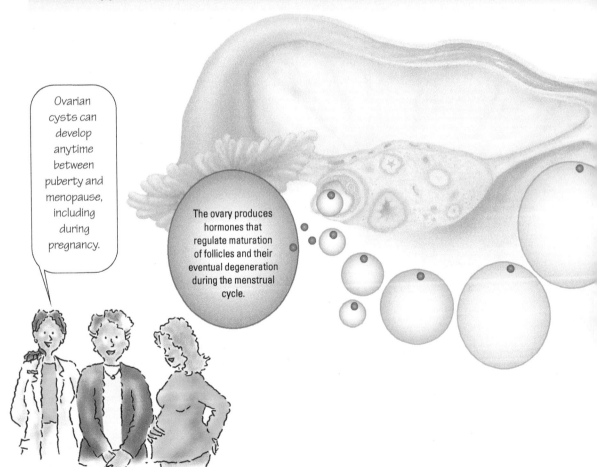

Ovarian cysts can develop anytime between puberty and menopause, including during pregnancy.

The ovary produces hormones that regulate maturation of follicles and their eventual degeneration during the menstrual cycle.

What to look for

- Breast tenderness
- Incomplete emptying of the bladder
- Fullness or heaviness in the abdomen
- Rectal or bladder pressure
- Dyspareunia (painful intercourse)
- Menstrual irregularities
- Pelvic or abdominal pain shortly before a menstrual period begins or just before it ends
- Nausea and vomiting

The corpus luteum eventually atrophies into the corpus albicans.

The follicular cyst eventually matures to a corpus luteum after ovulation and produces progesterone until the beginning of the next menstrual cycle.

During the proliferative phase of the menstrual cycle, many follicles develop but only one reaches maturity and produces estrogen.

When follicular development into a corpus luteum doesn't occur and the follicle continues to grow, an ovarian cyst can result. Two functional ovarian cysts may develop:
- Follicular cysts
- Luteal cysts

A dermoid cyst (or cystic teratoma) begins in the ovarian cell that forms into different tissue as the egg is fertilized and develops. This type of cyst can become very large and can contain hair, teeth, bone, and cartilage. It's most common in young women and during pregnancy.

Follicular cysts occur in the first 2 weeks of the cycle.

Corpus luteal cysts occur in the later half of the cycle.

Follicular cyst

Fallopian tube

Fimbriae

Opening of the fallopian tube

Semitransparent, distended, fluid-filled cyst

Follicular cyst of the ovary; the rupture of this thin-walled follicular cyst led to intra-abdominal hemorrhage.

Dermoid cyst

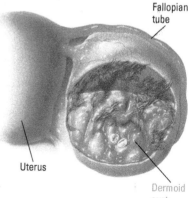

Fallopian tube

Uterus

Dermoid cyst

Prostate cancer

Prostate cancer is the most common cancer affecting men and the second cause of cancer death among men.

How it happens

About 85% of prostate cancers originate in the posterior portion of the prostate gland; the rest grow near the urethra. Adenocarcinoma is the most common form. Malignant prostatic tumors seldom result from the benign hyperplastic enlargement that commonly develops around the prostatic urethra in older men.

Slow-growing prostatic cancer rarely produces signs and symptoms until it's well advanced. Typically, when primary prostatic lesions spread beyond the prostate gland, they invade the prostatic capsule and then spread along the ejaculatory ducts in the space between the seminal vesicles or perivesicular fascia. Cancer cells can grow around the rectum and then travel to the vertebrae. When prostatic cancer is fatal, death usually results from widespread bone metastasis.

A closer look

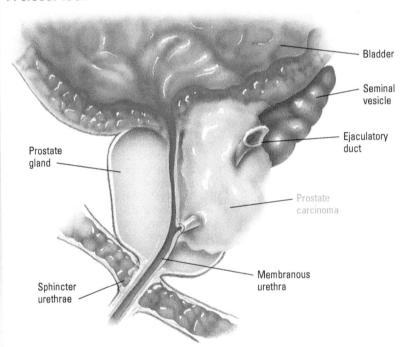

Prostate gland

Sphincter urethrae

Bladder

Seminal vesicle

Ejaculatory duct

Prostate carcinoma

Membranous urethra

What to look for

Prostate cancer seldom produces signs and symptoms until it's advanced. Signs of advanced disease are due to obstruction caused by tumor progression.
- Slow urinary stream
- Urinary hesitancy
- Incomplete bladder emptying and dysuria
- Frequency and urgency of urination
- Hematuria
- Erectile dysfunction
- Important to get a yearly digital rectal exam and PSA blood test

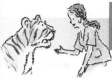

risky business

Risk factors for prostate cancer

- Age (more than 70% of all prostate cancer cases occur in men older than age 65)
- Diet high in saturated fats
- Ethnicity (Black men have the highest prostate cancer incidence in the world—more than twice that of White men. The disease is common in North America and northwestern Europe and is rare in Asia and South America.)
- Parent or sibling with the disease. The more individuals in a family who have the disease, the greater the risk for others in the family to develop it.

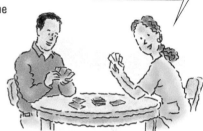

Remember to play your cards right...After age 50, you need to get yourself checked for prostate cancer every year.

Metastatic carcinoma

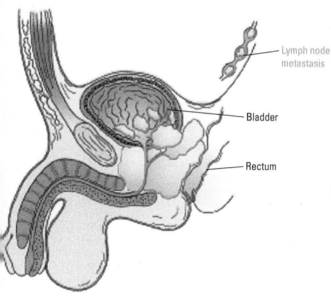

Lymph node metastasis

Bladder

Rectum

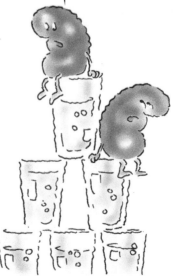

We may not be the cause of urinary problems when prostate cancer is involved. That prostate is stopping us from getting rid of all this water!

Testicular cancer

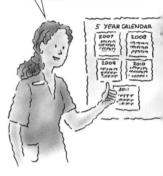

With the proper treatment, most testicular cancer patients survive way beyond 5 years.

Testicular cancer accounts for less than 1% of all male cancer deaths. The prognosis depends on the cancer cell type and stage. When treated with surgery, chemotherapy, and radiation, almost all patients with localized disease survive beyond 5 years. Testicular cancer is highly curable.

How it happens

With few exceptions, testicular tumors originate from germinal cells; about 40% become seminomas. These tumors, which are characterized by uniform, undifferentiated cells, resemble primitive gonadal cells. Other tumors—nonseminomas—show various degrees of differentiation.

Typically, when testicular cancer extends beyond the testes, it spreads through the lymphatic system to the iliac, para-aortic, and mediastinal nodes. Metastases affect the lungs, liver, viscera, and bone.

Are you saying that seminoma tumors look like us primitive cells?

A closer look

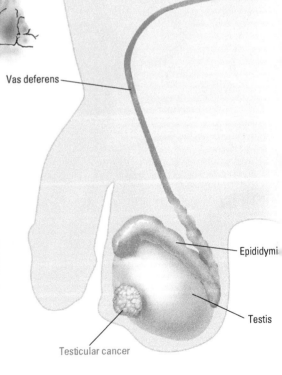

Vas deferens

Epididymi

Testis

Testicular cancer

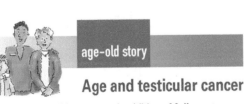

age-old story

Age and testicular cancer

Testicular cancer seldom occurs in children. Malignant testicular tumors are the most prevalent solid tumors in men ages 20 to 35.

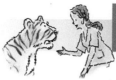

Risk factors for testicular cancer

Although researchers don't know the immediate cause of testicular cancer, they suspect certain contributing factors.

- Cryptorchidism (undescended testis), even when surgically corrected
- Family history (genetics)
- Ages 20 to 35 years
- Exposure to diethylstilbestrol (maternal)
- Infertility
- Ethnicity (The disease is rare in men who aren't white.)

Staging testicular cancer

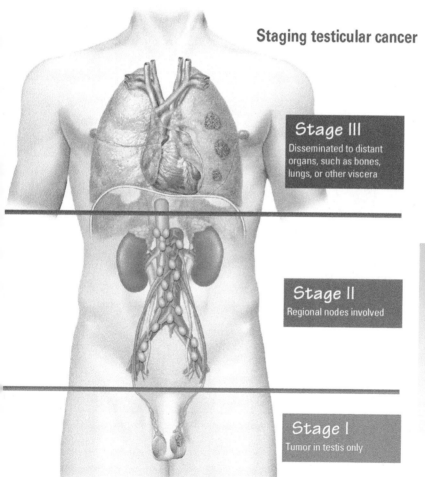

Stage III
Disseminated to distant organs, such as bones, lungs, or other viscera

Stage II
Regional nodes involved

Stage I
Tumor in testis only

What to look for

Early
- Heaviness or a dragging sensation in the scrotum
- Swollen testes
- Gynecomastia
- Painless lump in scrotum

Late
- Weight loss
- Cough
- Hemoptysis
- Shortness of breath
- Lethargy
- Fatigue

Uterine fibroids

Uterine fibroids, the most common benign tumors in women, are also known as *leiomyomas*. Uterine fibroids are tumors composed of smooth muscle and usually occur in the uterine corpus, although they may appear on the cervix or on the round or broad ligament. Uterine fibroids occur in 20% to 25% of women of reproductive age and may affect three times as many Blacks as Whites.

The tumors become malignant (leiomyosarcoma) in less than 0.1% of patients, which should serve to comfort women concerned with the possibility of a uterine malignancy in association with a fibroid.

> The true incidence of uterine fibroids is unknown because most women don't even know they have them.

How it happens

Leiomyomas occur from an overgrowth of smooth muscle and connective tissue in the uterus. A genetic predisposition exists. Both estrogen and progestin receptors are present in fibroids and elevated estrogen levels may cause fibroid enlargement.

During the first trimester of pregnancy, 15% to 30% of fibroids may enlarge and then shrink in the postpartum period. Some fibroids may decrease in size during pregnancy. Fibroids shrink after menopause, but some regrowth may occur if the woman begins hormonal therapy.

> Genetically speaking, some women are predisposed to uterine fibroids.

What to look for

• Abnormal or heavy menstrual bleeding (menorrhagia)
• Pain with menstruation (dysmenorrhea)
• Pelvic pressure

A closer look

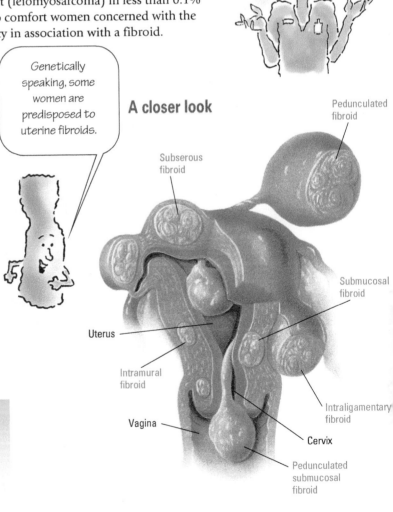

Pedunculated fibroid

Subserous fibroid

Submucosal fibroid

Uterus

Intramural fibroid

Vagina

Intraligamentary fibroid

Cervix

Pedunculated submucosal fibroid

Fibroid classification

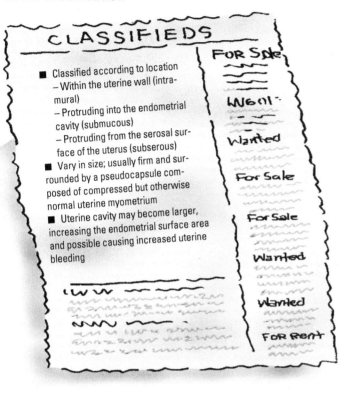

CLASSIFIEDS

- Classified according to location
  – Within the uterine wall (intramural)
  – Protruding into the endometrial cavity (submucous)
  – Protruding from the serosal surface of the uterus (subserous)
- Vary in size; usually firm and surrounded by a pseudocapsule composed of compressed but otherwise normal uterine myometrium
- Uterine cavity may become larger, increasing the endometrial surface area and possible causing increased uterine bleeding

Leiomyoma of the uterus

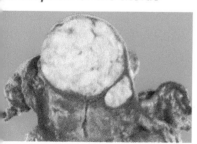

Fibroids compressing the bladder and rectum

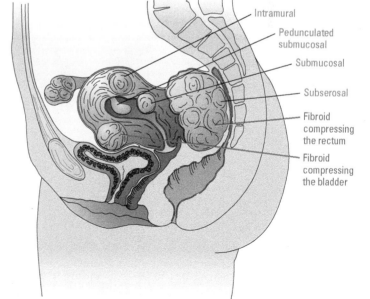

Intramural

Pedunculated submucosal

Submucosal

Subserosal

Fibroid compressing the rectum

Fibroid compressing the bladder

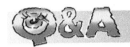

My word!

Solve the word scrambles to identify terms related to reproductive disorders. Then rearrange the circled letters from those words to answer the question posed.

In the illustration, label the anatomic structures involved in prostatic enlargement.

Question: Which reproductive disorder usually has a poor prognosis?

1. siapalrepyh ＿ ＿ ＿◯◯＿ ＿◯＿＿＿＿

2. oividng ◯◯＿＿＿◯＿

3. birofdi ＿＿＿◯＿◯＿

4. vasnievi ＿◯＿◯＿＿＿＿

5. llcurfoia ＿＿＿＿＿◯＿＿◯＿

6. rtaluestic ＿＿＿＿＿◯＿＿＿＿

Answer: ＿ ＿ ＿ ＿ ＿ ＿   ＿ ＿ ＿ ＿ ＿

1. ＿＿＿＿＿＿＿＿＿

2. ＿＿＿＿＿＿＿＿＿

3. ＿＿＿＿＿＿＿＿＿

4. ＿＿＿＿＿＿＿＿＿

5. ＿＿＿＿＿＿＿＿＿

6. ＿＿＿＿＿＿＿＿＿

Selected References

American Cancer Society. (2015). Testicular cancer. Retrieved from: http://www.cancer.org/cancer/testicularcancer/ overviewguide/testicular-cancer-overview-what-causes on February 23, 2015.

American Cancer Society. (2015). Endometrial (uterine) cancer. Retrieved from: http://www.cancer.org/cancer/ endometrialcancer/detailedguide/endometrial-uterine-cancer-key-statistics on March 17, 2015.

American Cancer Society. (2015). Uterine cancer. Retrieved from http://www.cancer.org/cancer/ovariancancer/ detailedguide/ovarian-cancer-risk-factors on March 12, 2015.

American College of Obstetricians and Gynecologists. (July 2014). Frequently asked questions. FAQ 163. Cervical cancer. Retrieved from: http://www.acog.org/~/media/For%20Patients/faq163.pdf

Buchanan, E. M., Weinstein, L. C., & Hillson, C. (2009). Endometrial cancer. *American Family Physician, 80*(10), 1075–1080.

Buckler, A., & Luu, P. (2013). Screening for ovarian cancer. *American Family Physician, 87*(10), 709–710.

Centers For Disease Control. (2015, March 31). Breast cancer. Retrieved from: http://www.cdc.gov/cancer/breast/ on March 31, 2015.

Crawford, P., & Crop, J. A. (2014). Evaluation of scrotal masses. *American Family Physician, 89*(9), 723–727.

Croswell, J., & Sikorski, C. (2011). Screening for testicular cancer. *American Family Physician, 84*(4), 451–452.

Croswell, J., & Shin, Y. R. (2013). Screening for prostate cancer. *American Family Physician, 87*(4), 283–284.

Croswell, J., & Costello, A. (2012). Screening for cervical cancer. *American Family Physician, 86*(6), 563–564.

Evans, P., & Brunsell, S. (2007). Uterine fibroid tumors: Diagnosis and treatment. *American Family Physician, 75*(10), 1503–1508.

McNicholas, T., & Kirby, R. (2012). Benign prostatic hyperplasia and male lower urinary tract symptoms. *American Family Physician, 86*(4), 359–360.

Roett, M. A., & Evans, P. (2009). Ovarian cancer: An overview. *American Family Physician, 80*(6), 609–616.

Schrager, S., Falleroni, J., & Edgoose, J. (2013). Evaluation and treatment of endometriosis. *American Family Physician, 87*(2), 107–113.

Trabert, B., Gruabard, B. I., Erickson, R. L., & McGlynn, K. A. (2012, March 27). Childhood infections, orchitis and testicular germ cell tumours: A report from the STEED study and a meta-analysis of existing data. *British Journal of Cancer, 106*(7): 1331–1334. Retrieved from: http://www.ncbi.nlm.nih.gov/pmc/articles/ PMC3314781/

Tria Tirona, M. (2013). Breast cancer screening update. *American Family Physician, 87*(4), 274–278.

U.S. Department of Health and Human Services. National Institute of Diabetes and Digestive and Kidney Diseases. (2014, September 24). Prostate enlargement: Benign prostate hyperplasia. Retrieved from: http://www.niddk. nih.gov/health-information/health-topics/urologic-disease/benign-prostatic-hyperplasia-bph/Pages/facts.aspx

Index

A

Acceleration-deceleration cervical injury, 78–79
  causes of, 78–79
  signs and symptoms of, 79
Acne, 228–229
  age as factor in, 229
  pathophysiology of, 228–229
  signs and symptoms of, 229
  types of, 229
Acquired immunodeficiency syndrome, 168–171
  children and, 169
  human immunodeficiency virus infection and, 168–171
  pathophysiology of, 168–169
  risk factors for, 171
  signs and symptoms of, 171
Acute coronary syndromes, 12–13
  pathophysiology of, 12
  risk factors for, 12
Acute coryza. See Upper respiratory tract infection
Acute infective tubulointerstitial nephritis. See Pyelonephritis
Acute renal injury, 208–209
  classifying, 208
  mechanism, 208
  phases of, 209
  signs and symptoms, 209
Acute respiratory distress syndrome, 48–49
  causes of, 48
  pathophysiology of, 48–49
  signs and symptoms of, 49
Acute tubular necrosis, 210–211
  causes of, 210
  pathogenesis, 211
  signs and symptoms, 211
Acute tubulointerstitial nephritis. See Acute tubular necrosis
Adaptive cell changes, 6–7
Addison's disease. See Adrenal hypofunction
Adrenal crisis, 188–189
  pathophysiology of, 188–189
  risk factors for, 189
Adrenal hypofunction, 188–190
  blocked secretion of cortisol in, 190
  forms of, 188
  pathophysiology, 188–189
  risk factors, 189
  signs and symptoms of, 190
AIDS. See Acquired immunodeficiency syndrome
Alcoholic cirrhosis, 106
Allergic rhinitis, 172–173
  age as factor in, 173
  allergen reexposure and, 173
  primary allergen exposure and, 172
  signs and symptoms, 173
Alzheimer disease, 80–81
  age as factor in, 80
  contributing factors for, 80
  risk factors for, 81
  signs and symptoms of, 81
  tissue changes in, 80
Anaphylaxis, 174–177
  age as factor in, 175
  complications of, 174
  pathophysiology of, 174–177
  risk factors for, 176
  signs and symptoms of, 176–177
Angina, unstable, 13
Ankylosing spondylitis, 178–179
  pathophysiology of, 178, 179
  signs and symptoms of, 179
  spinal fusion in, 178
Aortic aneurysm, 14–15
  age as factor in, 15
  pathophysiology of, 14
  risk factors for, 14
  signs and symptoms of, 15
  types of, 14
Aortic insufficiency, 37
Aortic stenosis, 38
Asthma, 50–52
  age as factor in, 50
  pathophysiology of, 50–52
  signs and symptoms of, 52
Atherosclerosis, 23, 199
Atopic dermatitis
  age as factor in, 180
  pathophysiology of, 180
  risk factors for, 181
  signs and symptoms of, 181
Atrophy, 6

B

Bacterial endocarditis. See Endocarditis
Bedsores. See Pressure ulcers
Benign prostatic hyperplasia, 248–249
  age as factor in, 249
  pathophysiology of, 248, 249
  risk factors for, 249
  signs and symptoms of, 249
Berry aneurysm, 83
Biliary cirrhosis, 106
Breast cancer, 250–251
  age as factor in, 250
  classifying, 250
  risk factors, 251
  signs and symptoms, 251
  staging, 251
  types, 250
Bronchopneumonia, 63
Burns, 230–231
  age as factor in, 231
  deep partial-thickness, 230
  full-thickness, 231
  pathophysiology of, 230
  superficial partial-thickness, 230

C

Cardiac tamponade, 16–17
  pathophysiology of, 16
  signs of, 17
Cardiogenic shock, 18
Cardiomyopathy, 19–22
  dilated, 19
  hypertrophic, 20–21
  restrictive, 22
Cardiovascular disorders, 11–43
Carpal tunnel syndrome, 130–131
  causes of, 130
  pathophysiology of, 130
  risk factors, 131
  signs and symptoms of, 131
Cell, 2–8
  adaptation, 6–7
  basics, 2–3
  division, 4–5
  injury to components of, 8
Cellulitis, 232–233
  age as factor in, 232
  pathophysiology of, 232
  risk factors, 233
  signs and symptoms of, 233
Cerebral aneurysm, 82–83
  age as factor in, 83